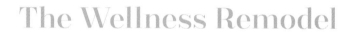

The Wellness Remodel

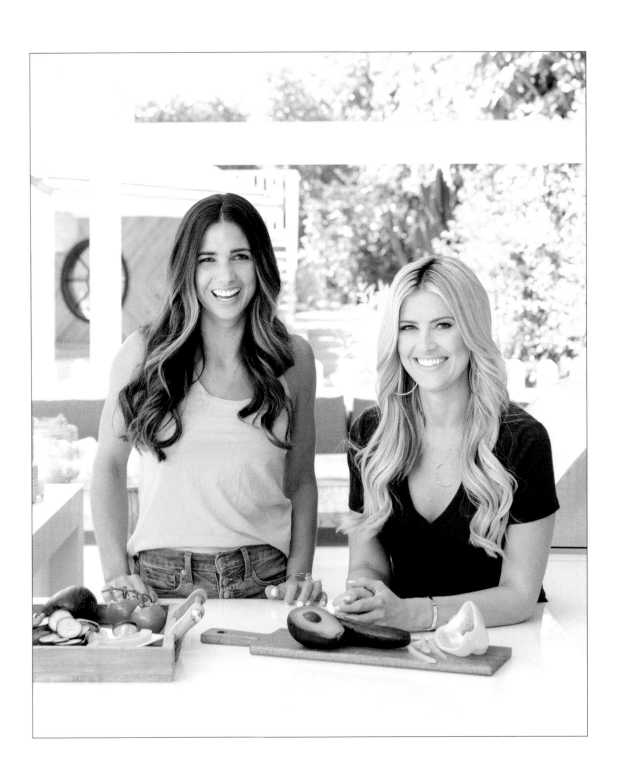

The Wellness Remodel

A GUIDE TO REBOOTING HOW YOU EAT, MOVE, AND FEED YOUR SOUL

Christina Anstead and Cara Clark

WITH RACHEL HOLTZMAN

HARPER WAVE

An Imprint of *HarperCollins*Publishers

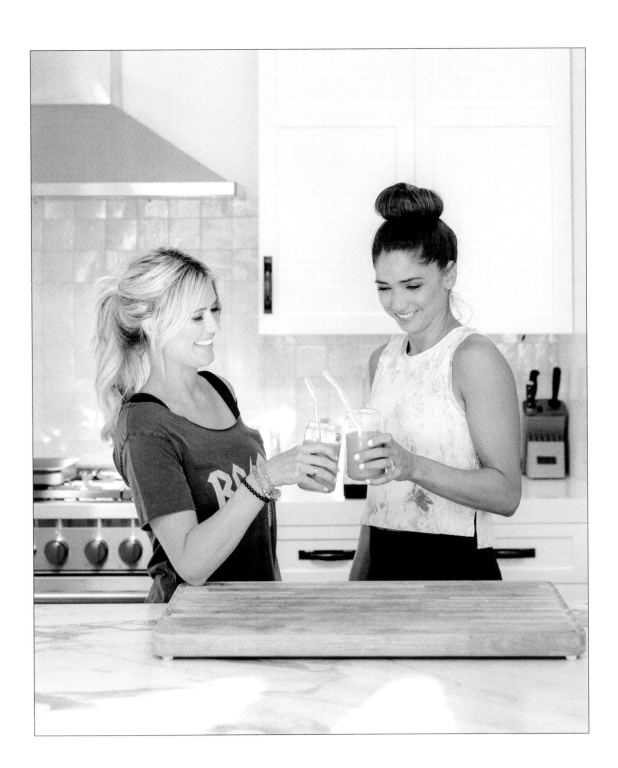

We dedicate this book to our readers

and their first steps on the path

to believing in themselves.

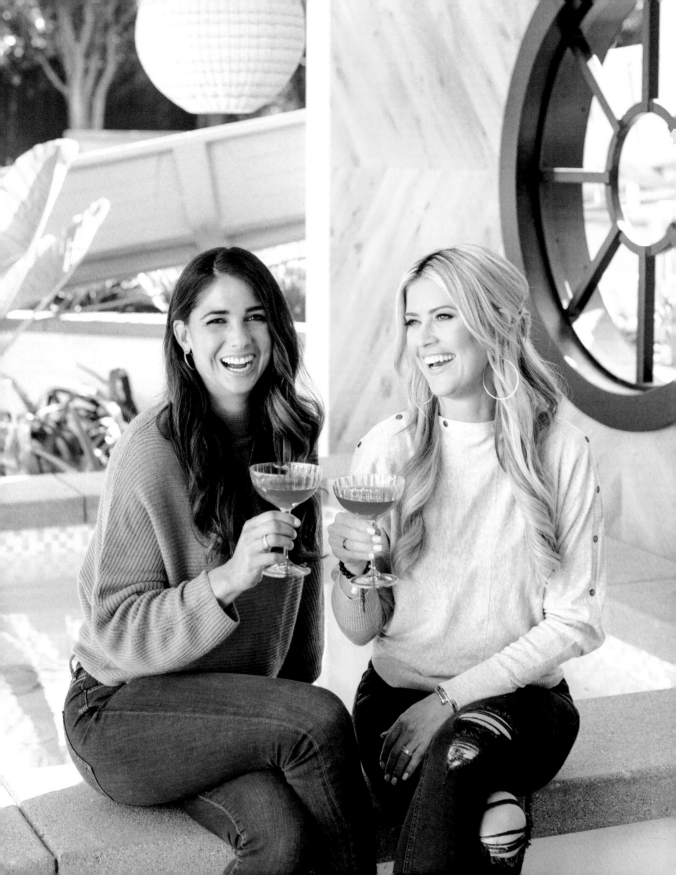

Contents

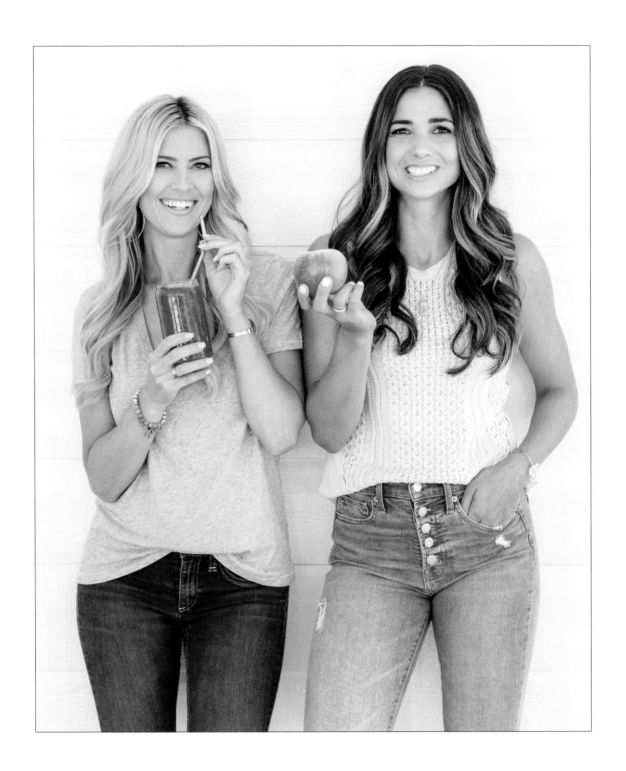

Part I

GUT
REHAB

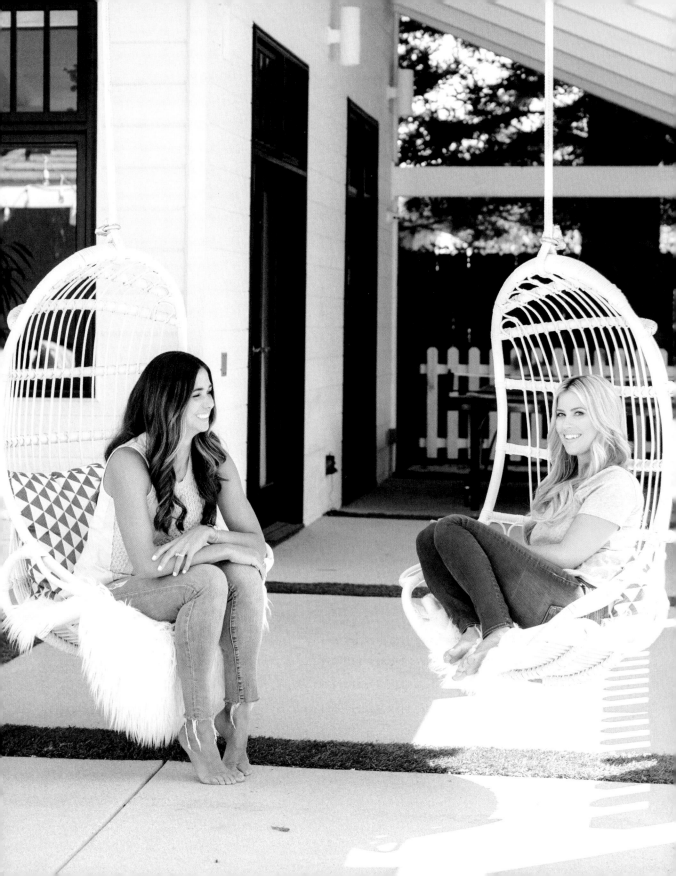

Chapter 1

WELCOME HOME

Christina: Anyone who knows me—or watches my HGTV shows *Flip or Flop* and *Christina on the Coast*—would probably use the same word to describe my life: BUSY. I work full-time (okay, who are we kidding, overtime) transforming not-so-amazing houses into incredible homes, plus hosting and filming the entire process, all the while keeping up with my three kids. And while I've spent seven years, eight seasons, and more than a hundred episodes making life look just a little more beautiful for the owners of my lovingly renovated and designed homes, I—like many women who are struggling to balance it all—haven't always been sharing that love with myself. I was over-caffeinating and under-eating. I lived on juices, protein bars, and coffee; and I was really scared of fats—any fats. On a daily basis my body felt sluggish, my brain was fuzzy, and bloating and indigestion were the norm. I attributed it to stress, but later found out that my symptoms were actually the result of two autoimmune disorders, Hashimoto's disease and polycystic ovary syndrome. I'm hardly alone when it comes to these issues—an estimated fifty million Americans suffer from autoimmune problems, and about 75 percent of them are women. So I know that a lot of you reading this can identify with what it feels like to struggle through each day, keeping fatigue and other symptoms at bay but not really thriving, focusing on taking care of everyone else, and putting your own needs last.

That's the reason I wanted to write this book. Ever since I first appeared on television, the number one question people have asked me has been, "How do you take care of yourself?" The reality is, for a long time, I didn't. But now I do. And while I've never really opened up about my health challenges before, my hope is that letting people into my life and sharing the tools I've used to transform my health can help improve the lives of other people struggling to feel their best. The most important thing I've learned on this journey is how to listen to my body—it seems so simple, but it's so easy to overlook. Your body is always talking to you. It knows what it wants and what it needs—you just have to learn how to listen.

This book is a compilation of all the lessons I've learned, distilled into one easy-to-read guide with advice that fits into any life, at any time. The way I've learned to approach diet (as in what I eat, not following a strict set of rules) and all the other elements of wellness that create a more balanced, healthy me doesn't actually take a lot of work. Because it's about a change in attitude and basic practices rather than some rigid, impossible-to-stick-to program, it can follow me everywhere, whether I'm at work, on vacation with my kids, out for a date night, or enjoying the holidays.

I'll include my personal regimen for how I've been able to eat, move, and breathe my way toward a healthier, more energized life. I promise that this is an anti-gimmick, anti-diet, pro-feeling-amazing book that reconnects you with real food in an approachable, sustainable way so that you can maintain a healthy weight without depriving yourself, fend off chronic illness or keep your symptoms at bay, and have a more even-keeled, peaceful relationship with the ups and downs of life. It's comprised of three main sections:

GUT REHAB: This is your new plan for eating *intuitively*. That means no fads, no all-or-nothing dieting, no off-limits food groups—just real food that makes your body look and feel like the best version of itself—and no rules other than learning how to tune in to your own hunger and craving cues. You'll hear a lot more about what you *should* eat rather than what you *shouldn't*. I'll walk you through the 14-Day Reset, our kickoff detox that will help you shed some of your negative eating habits, nourish the power center of your health (the gut!), and start creating a more energizing and wholesome sense of balance in your life. Once you've hit the "refresh" button, you'll be able to clearly hear what your body is asking for, and what doesn't make it feel so great. Remember, your body is your truest, most honest guide!

BUILDING A STRONG FOUNDATION: While eating a balanced, nourishing diet is the cornerstone to overall wellness, moving your body is a crucial piece, too. In this section of the book I'll share my secrets to finding an effective—and enjoyable—exercise routine that fits into an on-the-go life. No hour-long, high-intensity, punishing workouts required—thirty to forty-five minutes of even moderate movement is plenty to see results and get a hit of feel-good endorphins. Who has time for more than that, anyway?!

THE REWIRE: Finally, we'll discuss the most important element of all: reconnecting with your spirit and feeding your soul. I've experienced firsthand that your feelings can affect your physical body just as much as anything you eat. So it's important to work on your mental and emotional health in addition to your physical health. For me, faith and prayer combined with gentle yoga and meditation (we're talking ten to fifteen minutes before bed) does the trick; and I'll help you find whatever it is that grounds you, whether it's following a religious or spiritual practice, writing in a journal, or dancing around in your underwear (no judgment!).

Luckily, I have an incredible partner in wellness—and best friend—to help me with this mission. Cara Clark is pretty much the most awesome person I know. She manages to run her hugely successful businesses as a nutritionist and wellness coach while raising four kids—and kicks my butt at just about every workout we do together! Like me, she's a dreamer and a lover, and with her help, I was able to completely turn around not just my health but my whole life.

I met Cara in 2013, shortly after my ex-husband, Tarek, was diagnosed with thyroid cancer (now thankfully in remission), and I needed meal plans for his doctor-prescribed diet. Cara was super knowledgeable and support-ive, and she asked me about my own diet. At the time, I felt pretty confident that I was eating "good" food, but one look at my intake form and Cara had other ideas. She told me that I needed to start eating *more,* especially healthy fats and unprocessed carbs. She also suggested that I was *way* too stressed. We ended up meeting for breakfast one day, and it was clear from the moment we both ordered our triple-shot espressos that we had an instant connection. Our breakfast turned into a workout—she's one of the only people I know who loves doing the stairs at Thousand Steps Beach in Laguna as much as I do!—which turned into us becoming fast friends.

With Cara by my side I've learned how to look and feel my best by *adding,* not taking away. That translated into more food, more activities I enjoy, more laughter, more balance, and more peace. She truly helped me heal my body, mind, and spirit. And in this book, she'll be by my side once more, dishing out her signature no-nonsense advice on how to connect with the best ver-sion of you. But I'll let her tell you for herself!

Cara: What I noticed about Christina right off the bat—aside from our shared love of espresso and hard-core stair workouts—was that she needed some support for herself. Between caring for her sick husband, raising young kids, working around the clock, and—as we eventually learned—managing two autoimmune disorders, she wasn't nourishing herself properly. From the initial assessment she filled out for me, it was clear that she was under-eating—something I see in tons of my clients who think they're eating "healthy"—and that her stress was through the roof. It was a bad combination that was affecting her health, contributing to her feeling foggy and lethargic, and exacerbating the symptoms of her chronic conditions. I knew that we had to bring her cortisol (stress hormone) levels down and nourish her adrenal health, since the adrenal glands are responsible for producing hormones that help regulate metabolism, immune response, blood pressure, and other essential functions. To do that, I introduced her to my philosophy that starts—but doesn't end—with food. I explained that if she was serious about looking and feeling her absolute best and getting rid of her insomnia, digestive issues, and low energy, she was going to have to learn how the physical, emotional, and spiritual elements of her life all affect one another. We started by looking at her diet, and from there shifted focus to how she was moving her body, and last but not least, how she was caring for her mind. It's a process that takes time and practice, but with a few simple lifestyle changes, I promised that she could finally ditch some of her old damaging thinking and embrace a new set of health-promoting tools that she could reach for on even her busiest days. And that's exactly what we're going to teach you how to do in this book!

The Wellness Remodel is built from the very same guidelines and principles that I shared with Christina, which are the foundation of my practice as a nutritionist. My motto is: Real Food, Real People, Real Results. Because while I may work with celebrities and professional athletes in my practice, I want my programs to be accessible to everyone. Here are the basics:

• EAT MORE, NOT LESS: Because of the outdated thinking that calories in minus calories out equals weight loss, many people aren't eating enough food. One of the first things I worked on with Christina was getting her to consume more calories in the form of healthy fats, which would keep her feeling fuller longer. I also had her add healthy carbohydrates to her diet, like oats and quinoa—one of the key changes that ultimately helped resolve her PCOS and Hashimoto's symptoms. I'm also a big proponent of eating within an hour of waking up (sorry, intermittent fasters!) and every three to four hours thereafter to keep your blood sugar stable. Eating for stable blood sugar isn't just for people with diabetes—almost everyone can benefit from this strategy, as fluctuating glucose levels can result in fatigue, light-headedness, brain fog, and increased body-fat storage, as well as cravings for foods that don't serve our health (hello, processed sugar!). By eating frequently and combining macronutrients (carbohydrates, protein, and fat) at mealtimes, you can prevent glucose spikes, which in turn minimizes body-fat storage while combating many chronic diseases.

• EAT INTUITIVELY: One of the most important lessons that I hope you'll take away from this book is that food isn't the enemy. Carbs aren't the enemy; meat isn't the enemy; cheese isn't the enemy. I have clients who are afraid to eat fruit, thanks to recent fads like the ketogenic diet. Fruit is one of the most powerful foods that God gave us! I want you to understand that food is your friend and should deliver healing, not fear. Instead of filling this book with a list of "don'ts" or telling you that something is off-limits, we're going to let your body do that work for us. If something doesn't agree with your system (i.e., it causes bloating, indigestion, headaches, or any other discomfort), then that's for your body to tell you, not us. This is where the Reset comes in—to help you reboot your metabolism and get real clarity, in body and mind, about what serves you and what doesn't. For Christina, not eating meat causes her to feel tired and gain weight more easily, and eating dairy leaves her down for the count; while a serving of whole grains paired with a healthy fat gives her supercharged energy. Every body is different and there's no one-size-fits-all solution, but I promise we'll find the right solution for you.

• EAT FIVE COLORS A DAY: This is another great way to think about eating more food. I often find that people are hyper-focused on eating their greens and not getting in any of the other colors, including the beautiful jewel tones of fruit. We need all those powerful phytochemicals and micronutrients, plus all that beneficial fiber to feed and heal our gut—a topic we'll discuss in more detail soon. We also need at least 80 ounces of water a day. Get yourself a re-usable 40-ounce water bottle and fill it up once in the morning and once in the afternoon. The often-recommended 60 ounces a day just isn't enough to hydrate your organs and keep them functioning optimally, especially if you're active (working out regularly, on your feet at work, chasing kids around, etc.).

• MOVE FOR AT LEAST THIRTY MINUTES, FOUR DAYS A WEEK: That's it! No grueling hour-plus-long workouts. And it doesn't have to be high intensity, either. Walk your dog, play hide-and-seek with your kids, climb some stairs— that's minimally what your body needs to progress and excel. And if you want to work up to something more challenging, we've included some of our go-to workouts that we love to do together, as well as recommendations from some of our favorite trainers. People like to say that achieving physical transfor-mation is 80 percent what you eat and 20 percent how you move. But I say that you still need to be 100 percent of a person! And working out *does* matter—not only for how your body looks but, more important, how it feels.

• CELEBRATE YOUR SUCCESSES! When you feel good about what you're ac-complishing, you're more likely to set realistic goals for yourself. That's why

I always recommend tracking success by measures other than weight loss. Along this journey, I'll be asking you to check in with yourself regularly: Have your energy levels improved? How does your skin look? Do you feel more comfortable in your clothes? Are you feeling sharper and more focused at work? Are you able to be more present and patient with your family? These are all indications of health versus weight loss—and are all signs that you are on the right path.

● SET YOUR SPIRIT FREE: I believe that you can't fully heal or achieve your wellness goals until you strengthen your spirit. The same way you exercise your body, you need to work on the emotional and spiritual elements of yourself. Whether it's through meditating or attending a religious service, playing a musical instrument, journaling, practicing yoga, or any other mindfulness ritual, nourishing your spirit is the final piece of the puzzle that will help all the other areas of your life fall into place. For Christina, tending to her emotional health in addition to her physical health was the crucial part of her self-care regimen that helped her finally feel like herself again. On some days that might only look like fifteen minutes of Headspace (an amazing guided meditation app) before bed, and that's totally fine. A little attention to the spirit goes a long way.

Christina: When I started working with Cara, I thought, "This is the first program I've seen that actually *makes sense!*" There weren't any crazy gimmicks or complicated rules, just real food and plenty of it. It also didn't hurt that I finally felt good. Like, *really* good. I felt lighter in every sense of the word. I was clear and connected to a higher spiritual voice. Since my followers and Cara's clients have been begging us for our secrets to looking and feeling our best, and because we share the same philosophies about what makes for a well-rounded, fulfilling, and vibrant life, it just made sense that we do this project together!

In these pages, you'll find tons of tips and tricks for integrating healthy habits into your life, and it all starts with Cara's 14-Day Reset to help you refresh your connection with food, revitalize your gut health, and rev up the detoxifying functions of your bod. After you've figured out what foods work best for you, we offer a mix-and-match meal plan that takes into account the challenges of real life (including going out to eat or cooking for a family); our all-time favorite recipes (including desserts and cocktails!); and sample exercises and routines that don't require a gym.

The most important thing we want to communicate is that all of this information is intended to be helpful, customizable, and 100 percent doable. If it didn't pass the *Does this work for Christina's life?* test, it wasn't included in this book. Because—contrary to many people's opinions—when it comes to my health, I'm doing it all myself. From meal prep to workouts, I'm my own personal chef and trainer. So everything I do needs to be efficient, low-fuss, and, most important, effective—the same requirements that you most likely have, too! I want you to see that it's absolutely possible to be healthier and feel better, no matter how demanding your schedule. My hope is that by sharing this knowledge along with my own wellness journey—and Cara's, too—we can help you find your path. Every day that you wake up and choose to do things that nourish your body and spirit, every time you tune in to what you really, truly need to feel good, you're one step closer to building the strongest foundation possible for a long, healthy, fully charged life. Let's get started on this remodel!

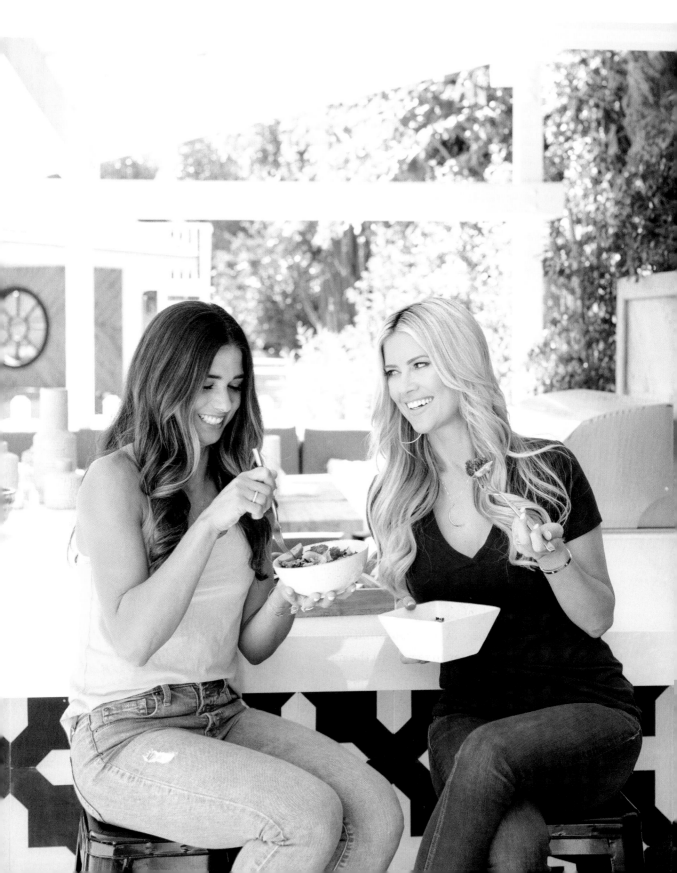

Chapter 2

YOUR BODY BLUEPRINT

Christina: For most of my twenties I remember feeling tired—like *exhausted*—pretty much all the time. Brain fog was a constant, and so was bloating. We're talking a pregnant-looking belly after meals. And speaking of pregnancy, when I eventually wanted to start a family but was having trouble getting pregnant, a test revealed that my body wasn't producing enough estrogen, and I had polycystic ovaries that weren't regularly releasing eggs. My doctor told me that the combination would make it difficult to conceive and carry a pregnancy to term—all the more a miracle that I was actually, unknowingly, pregnant with my daughter, Taylor, as I sat in her office. To be on the safe side, she prescribed me a progesterone supplement to help support the pregnancy. But because I'd managed to get pregnant, I didn't really think much about taking the hormone. I never stopped to ask any questions about how or why my body had become imbalanced in the first place.

After Taylor was born, I was back to the grind, constantly running on adrenaline, if I wasn't running on caffeine. I put myself through grueling high-impact workouts almost every day to stay in shape for filming, and it wasn't uncommon for me to skip meals—or just grab a protein bar or a juice and call it lunch—because when I get stressed, I lose my appetite. In my mind, I was living a "healthy" life: I was active and eating what I considered to be a good, "clean" diet. But when it started to take me a week to bounce back from a particularly tough workout, and I could barely make it through a day on set without feeling foggy and lethargic, I began to think something might be off.

Luckily, that's when God/the universe/fate sent me Cara. Within moments of going through my daily routine with her, she knew exactly what was going on: thanks to a steady diet of stress and intense workouts, my adrenal glands were worn out and not functioning properly. Cara explained to me that this control center is essential to optimal health because it produces hormones like cortisol (which regulates metabolism and your sleep rhythm), aldosterone (which helps control blood pressure), and adrenaline (which attunes your body's stress response). It turns out that if you're always operating in Code Red (which I definitely had been), then your body gets the message that it's always in a state of "fight or flight"—that caveman instinct we have to run away from danger or confront it. The problem is that this causes your adrenals to consistently pump out the stress hormones cortisol and adrenaline, which can cause an imbalance in other important hormones. The result: fatigue, body aches, anxiety, sleep disruption, and, for me, reproductive health issues. Cara also pointed out that I wasn't getting enough nutrients or eating often enough, which was causing my blood sugar to fluctuate too much and taxing both my immune system and brain health.

Cara suggested that the first and most important order of business was to establish a clean slate that we could work from, so I embarked on her 14-Day

Reset, which is a kind of full-body detox. We started by removing foods that tend to cause inflammation, like gluten, dairy, refined sugar, and processed foods. For a lot of people, these foods can trigger an immune response. While we want the body to bring out its big guns to fight off things that can make us sick, when it reacts to the foods we eat, a lot of harm can occur. Over time, an overactive immune response generates chronic inflammation that can have a damaging effect on just about everything—your gut, your brain, your heart, your lungs, your joints, and even your mood.

We also needed to restabilize my blood sugar by having me eat *more* food and *more* meals—especially meals that included fruits and vegetables along with a generous dose of healthy fats like avocados, nut butters, and olive oil. Eating this way kept my insulin levels in check and lessened my near-constant cravings for sweets.

But the most noticeable result of making all of these changes was that I suddenly had more mental and physical energy than I'd had in years. And yet it wasn't like any other "detox" I'd done before—there were no weird ingredients I had to track down at a health food store, and definitely no starvation or deprivation. My meals—all of which were completely eat-out-of-the-cup-holder, on-the-go friendly—kept me feeling satisfied all day long.

After two weeks, we slowly reintroduced foods we suspected might have been triggering my symptoms and monitored to see how my body reacted to them. That's when I discovered that I had a gluten intolerance—cutting out gluten had made a huge difference in how I felt and looked (no more bloated belly at the end of the day!), and when I reintroduced it, my symptoms came back right away. It was a major "aha!" moment about how my body would be my best guide when it came to figuring out what was right for it. It showed me so clearly that if I was going to take control of my health, then I was going to have to tune in and eat *intuitively*.

When I started listening to what my body wanted (plenty of fruit and vegetables and healthy fats) and what it didn't (gluten and red meat), it completely changed my relationship with food. I not only felt better than I ever had, I also saw more results than when I was counting every calorie and depriving myself of anything indulgent. Even with chocolate (daily), snacks (so many snacks), and cocktails (a girl's gotta kick back) in the mix—and even with dialed-down workouts, which we'll talk more about in part II—I was still feeling great in my clothes and in my own skin. This chapter is dedicated to helping you find the same relief and freedom that I found once I tuned out all of those old, damaging voices about what I *should* be eating and instead tuned in to the most powerful voice of all: mine!

But what really made me believe in Cara's program was when it was put to the test again. As you most likely know, your health isn't always a straight line, and that was definitely the case for me. After my son, Brayden, was born, I felt "off"—in more ways than could be attributed to the usual post-baby hormonal haze. During the pregnancy, my doctor had told me that my thyroid wasn't functioning "optimally" and put me on medication, but even that didn't seem to make a dent in the way I felt.

Desperate to find an answer, I turned to an integrative physician, who ran more complete thyroid bloodwork. We discovered from those tests that I also had Hashimoto's disease, which meant that my immune system was attacking my thyroid. That's a pretty big deal because your thyroid gland has some important jobs—like producing hormones that regulate brain and heart function, metabolism, and mood. I started reading everything I could find about Hashimoto's, and then suddenly it all clicked. I could see why I'd be feeling okay for a couple weeks, but then absolutely horrible and run-down for a week.

For a lot of people, this information would be overwhelming—and don't get me wrong, it was for me, too. But because I already had a clear line of communication with my body and because I understood how significantly my lifestyle choices could affect my health, I didn't have to start from scratch. I worked with my new practitioner to course-correct my medications, while also consulting with Cara to address what foods might be causing an immunogenic response (as in, making my immune system aggravated). I revisited the 14-Day Reset, this time paying close attention to how my symptoms would start to flare up when I added certain foods back into my diet. I started meditating in the evening and practicing yin yoga (we'll discuss this in more detail in chapter 7), which helped soothe the stress response in my body—a huge cause of inflammation. And Cara was always there for me with her friendship and laughter—some of the strongest medicine there is! With her support and with the insight I've gained into my own body's needs, I've been able to build a new baseline for my health, and I feel better than I ever have before (seriously, who says your twenties are the high point?!).

Cara: As Christina learned, lifestyle change isn't always easy, but there is great wisdom to be gained from listening to your body and shifting your choices to support its needs. Here's the thing: It is possible to feel like the strongest, most energetic, patient, tuned-in, vibrant version of yourself. It is possible to feel better than you ever have before. It all starts with making your health a priority.

On this program, that's just what you'll do. And you'll reap the rewards of treating your body right. The symptoms you once thought you had to live with because of genetics, chronic disease, or just plain life—headaches, brain fog, joint pain, imbalanced hormones, mood fluctuations, depression, anxiety, digestion issues, poor sleep, unwanted weight gain or loss, and so on—will dissipate. And yes, your clothes will fit better, too.

Am I going to carry you there on my back? Nope. *You* are going to get *yourself* there. Will this be the easiest thing you've ever done? Nope! But investing in your health is one of the best investments you'll ever make. And Christina and I will be with you every step of the way, giving you the tools and guidance you need. We can attest firsthand—as busy working moms who struggle every single day with making choices that support our health—that some very simple shifts can yield very meaningful results. All I ask is that you make a few changes to the way you're eating (and eventually, moving and thinking), which will give your body what it needs to start healing from the inside out. And in exchange, I promise that I'll *never* ask you to deprive yourself or do anything that makes your body feel bad. The goal here is to feel *good*.

The Program

The philosophy at the foundation of my work boils down to this simple formula:

STABLE BLOOD SUGAR → BODY RUNS OPTIMALLY →
INCREASED METABOLISM, ENERGY, AND FAT-BURNING

One of the things people love most about my program is that at its core there's really just one sensible and achievable goal: Eat for stable blood sugar. Every other "rule" or suggestion that you'll learn in this chapter leads back to that one objective, and the reasons for this are powerful but simple.

STABLE BLOOD SUGAR . . .
- Keeps your body burning stored fat (instead of lean muscle) for fuel
- Regulates your hunger hormones and reduces cravings
- Increases the available energy your body can use

When your blood sugar is stable, your mood will balance, your hormones can function as they should, your energy will increase, your memory and mental capacity will improve, your weight will settle into a healthy range, and your risk for blood sugar–related diseases such as metabolic syndrome, insulin resistance, diabetes, and heart disease will decrease. In short, you'll feel healthy, happy, and equipped with the clarity you need to live the life you want. Sounds pretty amazing. So how does it work?

The body gets glucose (aka blood sugar) from the food you eat, namely from carbohydrates. And the hormone insulin (produced by your pancreas) initiates and regulates the transport of glucose in your body. Most of the cells in your body use glucose for energy and other metabolic functions such as repairing and restoring tissues, transmitting and processing information, and keeping up with life's daily demands. Your brain also needs glucose in order to function optimally.

If **too much** glucose is present in the bloodstream, more insulin is released in response. There are two problems with this. First, when too much insulin is present all the time, your body becomes less sensitive to it, leading to a condition known as insulin resistance, or prediabetes. And second, all of that extra glucose gets stored as fat. Over time, chronic high blood sugar levels can also damage blood vessels, nerves, and organs and lay the groundwork for a variety of diseases, including autoimmune diseases.

If **too little** glucose is available in your blood, which is what happens when you follow a low-carbohydrate diet (I'm looking at you, keto!), then your liver hoards glucose so that your brain, which needs glucose to function, doesn't starve. While your body will start to break down fat to use as fuel, your brain can't run that way for long, and it will send out the Bat-Signal for more calories. That's the reason why when you skip a meal or go too long between meals, you find yourself running to the nearest donut or bag of chips. Your brain is hungry, and it wants glucose *now*!!

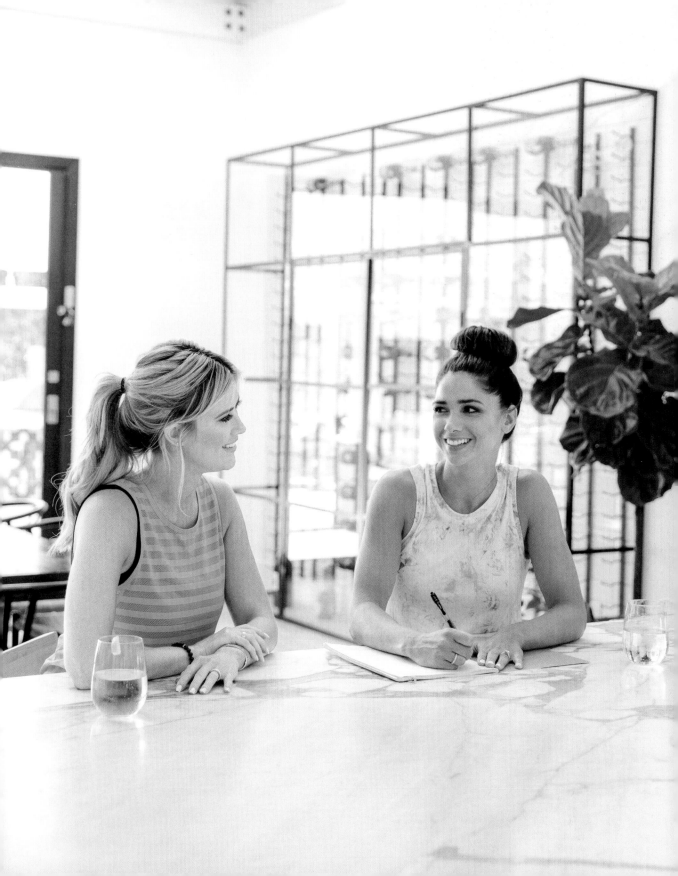

THE
5
GUIDELINES

The guidelines that make up the basis of this program are all focused on maintaining optimal glucose levels—preventing spikes that lead to weight gain and dips that lead to cravings and energy crashes. They are also designed to ensure that you're giving your body all the nutrients it needs for optimal health and longevity. Without further ado, here they are:

1. Eat a meal within one hour of waking up and every three to four hours after that. Try not to go more than four hours without eating.

2. Always pair a carbohydrate with a protein, fat, or both.

3. Eat four to five similar-sized meals throughout the day.

4. Eat five colors a day.

5. Be the expert on your body and listen to what it's telling you.

1

Eat a meal within one hour of waking up and every three to four hours after that. Try not to go more than four hours without eating.

Eating consistently throughout the day is the best way to ensure that your blood sugar never enters the drop-spike cycle. Instead, you'll reliably give your body fuel to keep it in the optimal fat-burning zone, where you'll feel the most energetic and clear-minded. Because of this, I recommend eating within one hour of waking up, give or take. I know that's bad news for the intermittent fasters out there, but I promise that you'll welcome the shift in your energy and appetite.

Intermittent fasting—or going for extended periods of time without eating—can actually shut down your hunger cues. Your body (specifically your gastrointestinal tract) is programmed to release the hormone ghrelin to cue you to eat, but intermittent fasting can decrease the amount of ghrelin in your system. While some people may see that as a good thing (less ghrelin = less hungry = eating less food), I beg to differ. If you're feeling less hungry, you're no longer inclined to eat small, frequent meals. This in turn slows your metabolism, disrupts your ability to maintain stable blood sugar, and also puts you in a position to burn glycogen from your muscles for fuel rather than stored fat. Also, when you shut down your body's natural inclination to signal that it needs more energy, you're shutting out the innate voice that tells you when your body needs nourishment and how much. That voice—as we'll discuss in more detail shortly—will help you relearn how to give your body exactly what it wants and needs. Plus, when you don't eat between dinner and breakfast, you're already reaping all the rewards of fasting! You're giving your body plenty of time to digest, heal, and rest—so you don't need to prolong the fast after you wake up. Eating during that first hour of the morning gently wakes your body and mind.

The *only* exception to this guideline is if you prefer to exercise in the morning. In that case, getting your heart rate up first thing is a great way to rev up your body, mind, and metabolism—so long as you're having a meal as part of your recovery.

WHEN FASTING IS PART OF YOUR FAITH

Many religions include a holiday that calls for fasting, and it always makes my clients a little bit nervous to veer from our program. But just as with everything else, I believe that anything done with good intentions can be beneficial, so I encourage them not to stress out about it. I also recommend taking the opportunity of a spiritual fast to focus on more than just *abstaining*. Think about *nourishment,* too—add a ten-minute meditation, a daily walk in the fresh air, five minutes in the morning to give gratitude for everything in your life that brings you joy (and even the things that don't!). Then, when your observance is over, go back to your routine, feeling refreshed and reenergized.

2

Always pair a carbohydrate with a protein, fat, or both.

In addition to vitamins, minerals, and water (aka micronutrients), your body also requires *macro*nutrients (aka "macros") in order to function optimally. These include protein, fats, and carbohydrates. Despite the bad rap that any of these essential nutrients has received in recent years, the fact remains that every single one of them is required if you want to live a long, healthy life. There are no bad guys here! Let's take a closer look at the players.

CARBOHYDRATES

PRIMARY FUNCTION IN THE BODY = ENERGY

Our body's preferred source of energy is carbohydrates—they literally fuel all of our metabolic functions (breathing, moving, digesting). Carbohydrates are necessary for digestion and absorption of both fats and proteins, and they break down into glucose in our bloodstream, which is used immediately as energy by our organs and every single one of our bodily systems (nervous, adrenal, endocrine, immune, etc.). Incidentally, the nervous system includes the brain, which is why getting enough carbohydrates is crucial for increasing mental focus and preventing fatigue.

I hope this comes as a pleasant surprise, since I'm guessing that a lot of you have been told at one time or another that carbs are the devil. Most of my clients—especially women—don't eat nearly enough carbohydrates because they've become so afraid of them. But omitting carbohydrates—including "resistant" starches in foods like potatoes, corn, and grains—can interfere with the function of the adrenal glands (affecting everything from mood to energy to fertility). That's because carbohydrates are the main source of glucose in your body, which provides you with immediate energy. Not getting enough carbs means that your body goes into starvation mode, which impacts the amount of cortisol you release. Both too much and not enough cortisol can stress out the adrenals, causing adrenal fatigue. But when you eat carbohydrates with healthy fats and proteins throughout the day, you can regulate these levels and reap all the physiological and emotional benefits.

One particular source of carbs that many of my clients have been told to avoid is fruit. While it is true that some fruits are high in sugar, the benefits of this miracle food far outweigh any dangers. Fruit is hydrating, nourishing, and packed with fiber and antioxidants—plus it's delicious. No healthy eating plan should require you to give up fruit!

Of course, I believe in all things in moderation, and that includes carbohydrates. When eaten excessively—or without a protein or fat—they can elevate your blood sugar and be stored as fat. So I offer a few rules of thumb when it comes to eating carbs.

Carbohydrate Rules of Thumb

Focus mostly on whole food, COMPLEX carbohydrates:

- Veggies and fruit (more on how to be mindful about fruit in a bit)
- Whole grains
- Beans/legumes (contain carbs, fat, and protein)
- Dairy (contains carbs, fat, and protein)

Limit SIMPLE carbohydrates:

- THE OBVIOUS: soda, candy, sweets, and processed foods such as chips, cookies, crackers, and other packaged items
- THE SNEAKY ADDED SUGARS: Many packaged and prepared foods—and those touted as "health" products like green juices and energy bars—contain sneaky sugar replacements like brown rice sugar, malt syrup, and high-fructose corn syrup.

FATS

The low-fat movement of the '90s gave fat a bad reputation that still persists—so many of my clients, like Christina, are nervous about eating too much fat. So let me share with you what I share with them: Fat is nothing to fear! In fact, getting enough fat is essential to your health.

Our most concentrated form of energy in the body is dietary fat. As it is oxidized by the body, fat yields more than *three times* the amount of energy compared to amino acids (from protein) or glucose (from carbs). Fat also plays an important role in absorbing certain vitamins—such as A, D, E, and K—and helps slow the secretion of hydrochloric acid in the stomach, which prolongs the emptying time and creates a longer-lasting feeling of fullness after a meal. And our circulatory, lymph, immune, and nervous systems rely on healthy dietary fats, namely because they help transmit messages in the body from one system to the next, protect nerves and organs, and manufacture disease-fighting antibodies. Oh, and it doesn't hurt that fatty acids are the building blocks of healthy cell membranes, which contribute to youthful, supple-looking skin!

Food Sources of Healthy Fat
ANIMAL SOURCES

- Dairy
- Some lean meats (venison, bison, chicken and turkey breast, pork tenderloin), wild-caught fish and seafood
- Eggs

- Plant-derived oils (olive, grapeseed, sunflower, safflower, avocado)
- Avocados
- Nuts and seeds

LEARNING NOT TO FEAR FAT

Christina: My generation came of age at a time when everyone was freaking out about fat. Low-fat diets and food products were all the rage (anyone else remember those low-fat cookies?). I was fully convinced that if I wanted to lose weight, I needed to avoid all fat. I'd always been fine with carbs (okay, total understatement—Cara told me that I ate like a toddler because I was always snacking on crackers, pretzels, and chips!), but fat was pretty much off-limits. I would carefully measure out one little scoop of peanut butter for the day, and there was a lot of lean turkey and grilled chicken breast in my life. But one of the first lessons Cara taught me was not to fear fat. I had to ease into the idea, but after I got accustomed of eating more fat than I ever had—especially peanut butter, avocado, and salmon—I saw firsthand that it was one of the missing pieces for me having as much energy as I needed during the day. And I learned that *everything* tastes better with a schmear of something rich and creamy (whether it's nut butter, hummus, egg, avocado, or cheese) and that eating more fat definitely doesn't make you fat—just satisfied!

PROTEIN

PRIMARY FUNCTIONS IN THE BODY = GROWTH, MAINTENANCE, AND REPAIR

Unlike carbs and fat, protein has maintained its positive reputation in the wellness world. However, there are arguments about whether it's optimal to get your protein from animal sources or plant sources. The reality is both plant and animal proteins offer health benefits. So long as you're getting enough protein every day—and you actually don't need a ton!—the sources are up to you. Protein plays a vital role in the maintenance and development of all regulatory and structural components in the body. It provides the primary building blocks for muscles, blood, nails, hair, and organs like the skin, heart, and brain. It's also required for the production of enzymes and hormones that regulate a variety of bodily functions, such as reproduction, muscle growth, and metabolism. If your body has to rely on protein for energy (versus fats or carbohydrates), then it is depleting the nutrients it needs to perform these essential functions.

Food Sources of Protein

ANIMAL SOURCES

- Lean meats (chicken and turkey breast, pork tenderloin)
- Wild-caught fish and seafood
- Eggs
- Lean game meat (venison, bison)

PLANT SOURCES

- Beans/legumes (lentils, peas, black/white/navy/pinto/red beans, chickpeas, soy/edamame)
- Nuts (almonds, cashews, pistachios, pecans, walnuts, Brazil nuts)

- Seeds (pumpkin, sunflower, hemp, chia, flax)
- Quinoa
- Some amounts in whole grains (oats, brown rice, bulgur, barley, farrow, whole grain pastas, etc.)
- Small amounts in certain veggies like dark leafy greens (but not enough to stand alone as a protein source)

COMBINING MACRONUTRIENTS

What I've learned from years of listening to my own body and observing those of my clients is that it's not only *what* we eat but also *how* we eat it. I've seen time and time again that giving the body carbohydrates paired with slightly smaller portions of protein and fat is the sweet spot that most of our bodies crave. When you combine your carbohydrates with fat and protein, you will burn fat for fuel all day long. When you eat (roughly) the correct ratios of carbohydrates, fat, and protein, you experience healthy energy and brain function. And when you eat the proper amount of all of these macronutrients, you avoid vitamin and mineral deficiencies. Sold yet?!

In general, a good balance to aim for at each meal is:

- 50 percent of calories from carbohydrates
- 30 percent of calories from fat
- 20 percent of calories from protein

That said, I'm not necessarily advocating that you count your calories (which we will discuss in much more detail soon). I'm also not recommending that you need to apply this as a hard-and-fast rule. That's because every body is different, and your body's needs will shift every day and with every meal. Use these numbers as guidelines and then go by how you feel.

3

Eat four to five similar-sized meals throughout the day.

Keeping your body consistently fueled throughout the day with balanced, nourishing meals is the most effective way to keep your blood sugar stable. And when I say eat four to five meals a day, I mean *meals*. On average, most women need between 1,600 and 1,800 calories a day. While I'm not suggesting that you count every calorie, I do think it's a helpful tool to understand just how much food we're talking about here. And the beauty of kicking off this program with the 14-Day Reset is that you'll start to get a feel for your ideal meal size. When I began working with Christina, the biggest challenge I faced was getting her to eat *more*. She went from taking in about 300 calories a meal to 400 to 500! But before you slowly back away from this book and head to the nearest juice cleanse, consider this: Your body needs fuel—especially if you're out there working your butt off every day (I see you #MotherHustler!). Ever tried running a car with no gas in the tank? Your body is no different—if you run it on empty for too long, things start to break down. As I like to say, "Your body keeps score . . . and it always wins."

Christina: One of the first things Cara did when we started working together was to suggest that I eat more food. Between a crazy schedule on set, running around with my kids, and generally believing that I needed to limit how much food I ate in order to be in camera-ready shape, I'd gotten into a food routine that was pretty minimal. But Cara helped me see that I was actually depriving my body of energy and making it work way too hard to get what it needed, which was aggravating my autoimmune symptoms and making me feel sluggish and foggy.

Cara promised that if I added more food I wouldn't bulk up. So breakfast went from a protein bar to overnight oats or a rice cake with peanut butter and sliced banana on top. I swapped green juices for smoothies, or at least added some protein on the side if I still wanted juice. Instead of a basic sandwich with hollowed-out bread, lettuce, tomato, and turkey breast, I started digging into giant salads with all the stuff—salmon, avocado, beans, tomato, hard-boiled egg, blue cheese crumbles, you name it. Or an English muffin with turkey bacon, avocado, and a sunny-side-up egg (pretty much my pregnancy go-to!). I also started eating more legumes, and a big, hearty pot of chili has been on rotation pretty much every week since. I noticed a difference almost right away—I had *so* much more energy, I didn't gain any weight, and best of all, I wasn't making my life more complicated because all of these meals were so easy to make and super portable.

Cara: The idea of eating more to lose weight doesn't make sense to a lot of people—especially the women in my practice. Most of the ladies I've worked with have had a difficult time escaping the pervasive message of our diet culture, which is all about restricting calories. This is unfortunate because calorie restriction leads to lethargy, headaches, cravings, negative self-talk, and the risk of health problems due to nutrition deprivation. I also tell my clients that when they restrict, yes, they will become a smaller version of themselves. But they won't be targeting the fat that accumulates in the places they usually don't want it to (butt, upper legs, belly, arms, etc.). Eating less food doesn't do any favors for body composition, since the body starts to burn calories from muscle instead of fat. But most of all, calorie restriction isn't sustainable! It does nothing to break the cycle of restricted/disordered eating that's been ingrained in so many of us, and it definitely doesn't set you up for long-term success—or happiness.

THE ONE TOOL YOU WON'T NEED: A SCALE

Christina: I haven't stepped on a scale since 2013. In my twenties, I cared so much about what I weighed, but when I got serious about nutrition and learned to trust my inner voice about whether I was nourishing myself properly, I stopped caring about that number. For me, it's so much more about how I feel, how I'm moving, and how my clothes fit.

So one of the first things I recommend when starting this process is not checking the scale. You're going to be drinking more water, eating more plant-based carbs (which carry more water), and moving your body in a way that protects your muscle instead of burning it for fuel. For some people, that might not initially translate on the scale. Instead, go by how you feel. If you're feeling more vibrant, if your mood feels more stable, if you're getting out of bed more easily in the morning and winding down more smoothly at night, and you just feel GOOD, you're not necessarily going to see that on a scale. Of course, you can also use how your clothes fit as a gauge, or you can occasionally take your measurements (chest, waist, hips, thighs, and arms). That's a great way to see how you're actively losing fat from the places where you tend to store it.

4.

Eat five colors a day.

The fourth pillar of my philosophy is making sure that you're getting most of your carbohydrates from five colors a day, meaning from whole-food fruit and vegetable sources. It could be green, blue, yellow, orange, white, brown, or red—just make sure they're mostly unprocessed (meaning they don't come in a box, bag, or bottle or contain additives). The reason this guideline deserves a spot on the list is because fruits and veggies get their individual characteristics like color, smell, and texture from special disease-fighting, body-healing compounds called phytochemicals. So the greater the variety of plants you eat, the greater the variety of benefits you get, such as reducing inflammation, boosting collagen production, strengthening the immune system, lowering blood pressure and cholesterol, improving brain and heart health, and even fighting cancer. Plus, eating all these plants helps to promote good digestion (thanks, fiber!), and, most important, helps heal and support the gut.

You've probably heard about the "gut," or the microbiome, because it's been one of the most talked-about topics in wellness circles in recent years. I won't give you a full-on Biology 101 lesson here, but what you need to know is this: Your gut and its community of diverse, beneficial bacteria is the center of your health. Seventy percent of your immune cells live in your gut, and 95 percent of your serotonin—the feel-good hormone that helps promote feelings of well-being and happiness—is produced there. That means that your body's ability to fend off illness and disease and regulate your moods is in large part dictated by the huge community of beneficial bacteria that call your gut home. These bacteria—six pounds of them, to be exact—thrive when we thrive. Meaning they are stronger and more resilient when they're fed a steady diet of fiber from a diverse range of whole-plant foods and probiotic-rich foods like yogurt or kimchi, and get enough exercise and sleep.

However, when these bacteria don't get the nutritional love they need or they're forced to compete with the bad bacteria introduced by artificial sweeteners or too much alcohol, processed sugar, and saturated fat—or the lining of the gut itself is damaged by inflammation, typically because of an immune response to foods such as gluten or dairy—then you start to see the effects in your health. An unhealthy microbiome can result in digestive issues (bloating, diarrhea, and constipation), skin eruptions (acne and eczema), mood disorders (anxiety and depression), suppressed immunity, chronic illness, and autoimmune disease.

The great news is that it's easy to take care of your gut and the microbes that call it home. The 14-Day Reset is meant to give your gut a break from any foods that might be irritating it or depleting your microbes, as well as help you identify what those foods are so you can consider removing them from your diet over the long term. And your good-guy bacteria are happiest when they're fed a fiber-rich diet filled with whole foods, especially plants and resistant starches. So hitting your five colors is basically giving your gut an all-you-can-eat wellness buffet.

EAT A RAINBOW EVERY DAY!

RED

Beets	Pink and red grapefruit	Red apples	Red potatoes
Blood oranges		Red bell peppers	Rhubarb
Cherries	Pomegranate	Red chiles	Strawberries
Cranberries	Radicchio	Red grapes	Tomatoes
Guava	Radishes	Red onions	Watermelon
	Raspberries	Red pears	

ORANGE/YELLOW

Apricots	Mango	Rutabaga	Yellow apples
Butternut squash	Nectarines	Summer squash	Yellow pears
Cantaloupe	Oranges	Sweet corn	Yellow peppers
Carrots	Papaya	Sweet potatoes	Yellow potatoes
Golden beets	Peaches	Tangelos	Yellow tomatoes
Golden kiwi	Persimmons	Tangerines/ clementines	Yellow watermelon
Grapefruit	Pineapple		
Lemon	Pumpkin	Winter squash	

GREEN

Artichokes	Brussels sprouts	Green beans	Leafy greens
Arugula	Celery	Green bell peppers	Leeks
Asparagus	Celery root	Green chiles	Limes
Avocado	(celeriac)	Green grapes	Okra
Bok choy	Chayote squash	Green onions	Snow peas
Broccoli	Cucumbers	Green pears	Sugar snap peas
Broccoli rabe	Endive	Honeydew	Watercress
Broccolini	Green apples	Kiwi	Zucchini

BLUE/PURPLE

Blackberries	Plums	Purple carrots	Purple and black
Blueberries	Purple and black	Purple cauliflower	figs
Eggplant	grapes	Purple endive	Purple grapes
	Purple cabbage		Purple potatoes

WHITE/BROWN

Bananas	Jerusalem	Mushrooms	Turnips
Brown pears	artichokes	Onions	White corn
Cauliflower	(sunchokes)	Parsnips	White nectarines
Garlic	Jicama	Potatoes	White peaches
Ginger	Kohlrabi	Shallots	

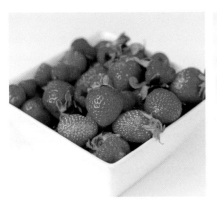
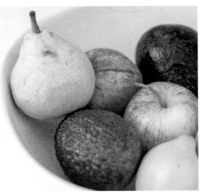
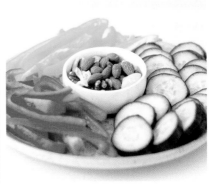

5

Be the expert on your body and listen to what it's telling you.

All of the guidelines in this book support a more mindful approach to eating, otherwise known as "intuitive eating." The goal of intuitive eating is to follow your body's cues and respond to them in kind—eating when you're hungry, eating enough to feel full, eating the foods that make you feel your best, and choosing not to eat foods that leave you feeling unwell. In the process, you'll be able to take the anxiety and guesswork out of eating and build a healthier relationship with your food, mind, and body.

I've found that by helping people tune in to their bodies, they begin to trust themselves. Because when you learn how to decipher what your body is telling you, when you can tell that a particular food is or isn't what your body needs to function optimally, and when you know what it actually *feels like* to feel your best, it will be easy to make decisions about what, when, and how to eat. That journey is all about your wisdom, not mine. This is also why I don't categorize any foods as off-limits and why I don't recommend calorie counting. There are no such thing as "bad" foods, only foods that make us feel bad—and those foods are different for everyone.

If you're doing this program with a partner, there's a good chance that the two of you will end up with meals that look different based on your unique physiological needs. Christina can't go a morning without her overnight oats, but oats make me feel bloated. I love going big on avocado in my salads, but too much fat in a meal makes Christina want to curl up and take a nap. And we both agree that gluten leaves us feeling terrible, but I have plenty of clients who thrive on diets that include gluten. So I don't believe in eliminating entire food groups or nutrients just because of my own intolerances or even what the nutritional science world is telling me. Because nutritional science, like any science, is always evolving. At the end of the day, you know your body better than any nutritionist.

The same logic applies to my advice about how many calories you need in a day. I offer guidelines because most people underestimate how much they should be eating, but the fine-tuning is up to you. The key thing to remember is that the literal definition of a calorie is a unit of fuel. So on days when you need more fuel—you go for a strenuous workout, you're barely sitting down between your kids' activities, or you're just feeling hungry—by all means give your body that sustenance. The alternative is sending your body into a low blood sugar cycle, leading to cravings, fatigue, and burning muscle instead of fat. I'd much rather you went for the extra serving of veggies and hummus!

RESET AND REUNITE

The best way to quiet all the noise about what you "should" or "shouldn't" eat and get reacquainted with your inner wisdom is to commit two weeks to the 14-Day Reset. By following a meal plan and eliminating any potential food intolerances, you'll hit the refresh button on your metabolism, restoring your gut health and building a strong foundation for moving forward with the rest of the program. During these two weeks you'll also give your body a break from potential allergens, such as gluten and dairy, as well as inflammatory foods like processed sugar and alcohol (temporarily!). Once you've completed the Reset and have gained some clarity on how your body feels after each meal, you can begin reintroducing these foods one by one. As you monitor how you feel, you'll know right away whether they're serving you or not.

Now let's get going and start to reset your health!

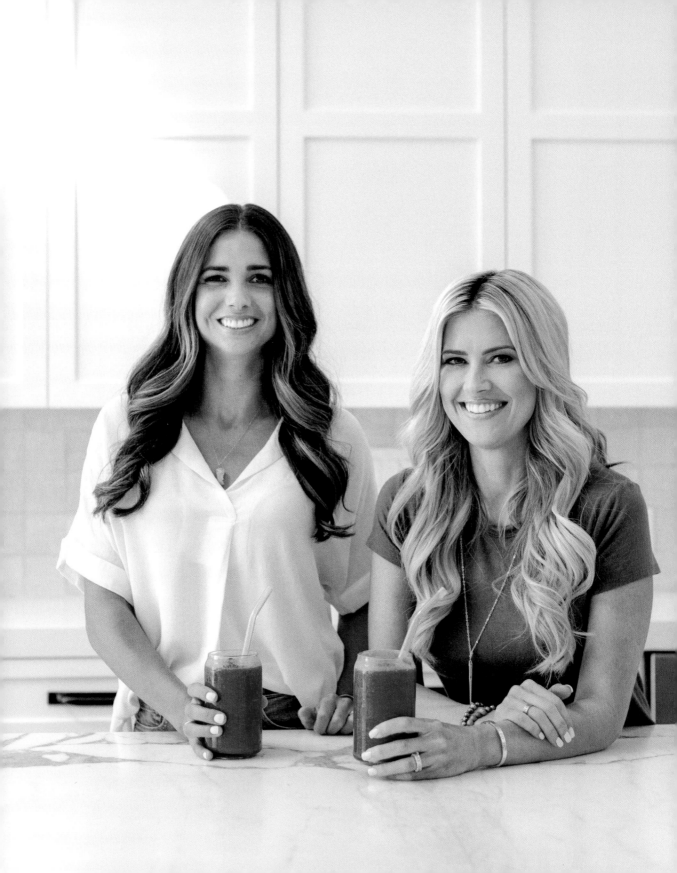

Chapter 3

START WITH A
BLANK SLATE

Christina: If you're anything like me, you might be a little anxious about going on a detox for two weeks. I still remember how I felt when Cara first told me that I had to give up certain foods—especially sugar and alcohol. I mean, really? I wasn't exactly pumped. But I also knew that I wasn't feeling great. My autoimmune symptoms weren't completely managed by medication, and I felt bloated and foggy. So I gave Cara's protocol a shot, and within a few days, I felt *amazing*. Seriously—my digestive system completely rebooted, my stomach no longer felt distended after every meal, and my energy shot through the roof. But I was most surprised to find that at no point during the process did I feel hungry or deprived. I had tons of options to choose from, like fruits and vegetables (obviously); fish, lean meats, and beans (give me a huge salad with these on top and I'm the happiest girl ever); plus nuts and nut butters. Then, when it was time to slowly reincorporate the foods I'd eliminated from my diet, I was surprised at how clearly I could feel my body telling me that some of them just didn't get along with my system. Red meat? Bye. Butter? Nope. Fried foods? See ya. Was I sad to say goodbye? A little bit, sure, but once I knew how great I could feel, I didn't want to go back. Of course, I do still enjoy the occasional indulgence, but I'm telling you right now: Not feeling well after you eat something kinda makes it not worth the splurge.

Now I actually look forward to the occasional detox. If I'm on the road and don't have access to healing, nourishing food or I'm eating handfuls of chips all day, it's the perfect time to hit the reset button. Or if I'm starting to feel run-down or notice an uptick in my autoimmune symptoms, I can do Cara's reset to help me pinpoint what's triggering my flare-up. Sometimes the suspect isn't an entire food group or a type of food that's typically reactive. For me, eating too many nuts and nut butters or even "healthy" snack bars can throw my digestive system out of whack. By detoxing, I can see exactly how my body responds to these foods in a way that's perfectly tailored to me. When you try out this 14-Day Reset, you, too, will be able to connect with what makes your body feel uniquely amazing. Good luck!

Cara: Whether you're hoping to finally ditch the diet script, shed a few pounds, boost your energy levels, tone up, or just discover some new healthy meal ideas, these next two weeks are going to lay the foundation for a lifetime of feeling good. Still need convincing? Here are a few of the benefits you'll get from the Reset:

- Reduced fat storage and increased energy
- The ability to identify food intolerances or sensitivities
- A healthier relationship with food
- A reset palate so it can better appreciate the flavors of real food

During the next fourteen days, you can expect a lot to happen. You'll finally feel in control of your eating decisions; you'll feel a balancing effect in your mood; you'll experience a boost in energy and mental clarity; and you'll be confident and comfortable in your own skin. Will you lose weight? Absolutely. Because you'll be revving your metabolism while allowing your body to let go of unnecessary fat storage, you'll notice in the first few days that your clothes are fitting differently. But is that the main goal? Not necessarily.

Any time you're making a big change in your life, it's important to connect with *why* you're doing it. I strongly encourage you to write down a list of the reasons that are motivating you to make these positive changes in your life—more than trying to fit into a dress for that wedding next month or looking great for a beach vacation. Dig deep—what do you really want? How will regaining your health or feeling better in your own skin affect your life? Christina and I both gave ourselves the challenge of connecting with our whys, and here's what they looked like:

Cara's Whys:
1. My body is a temple, only given to me as loan. I need to honor it and I want to teach my kids the same.

2. Eating right gives me the energy to play more!

3. I want to have FEWER mood swings and MORE patience for the constant "spilled milk" episodes. (Hypothetically.)

4. I love overhearing my three-year-old tell her friends "my mama says it's healthy."

5. My life isn't just about me! It's dedicated to helping others, supporting my children, and being a strong partner to my husband.

Christina's Whys:

1. Eating well is one thing I can control, unlike how many hours of sleep I'm going to get (or not) or how much time I'll have to exercise.

2. I want to feel and see the difference from my workouts. I don't have a lot of time to get them in, and I know they're enhanced by what I eat!

3. When my head starts spinning with all the things I need to get done, I want the energy and focus to stay in the game.

4. Because I feel so proud when my kids ask me for avocado!

5. So I can avoid the doctor. Fewer flare-ups equal fewer visits.

Getting Started

In the pages that follow, you'll find the day-by-day breakdown of the 14-Day Reset. We've included meal plans, instructions, tips, and even weekly grocery lists to help you get organized. Basically, we've done the legwork for you so all you need to do is shop, eat, and enjoy!

GUIDELINES AND TIPS AT A GLANCE

WHAT TO EAT:

- Whole foods, or foods as close to their natural state as possible: fruits and vegetables, lean animal proteins, nuts, seeds, legumes, and healthy fats. Choose organic whenever possible.

- Carbs from natural sources: fruits, veggies, legumes, and whole grains.
- Fats from healthy oils (coconut, olive), nuts, seeds, dairy, and avocados.
- Lean protein. Think chicken, eggs, fish, and turkey for animal sources, or legumes/beans for vegetarian options.
- Meals including one fat, one protein, and two carbs (perhaps a grain and a veggie).
- A variety of colors (minimum of five per day).
- Spices and fresh herbs to add flavor to foods. If you need a little salt, be sparing and use pink Himalayan salt, as it contains beneficial trace minerals.
- Plenty of water: at least half your body weight in ounces per day. Drink at least 16 ounces before breakfast, with every meal, during and after exercise, and sip throughout the day.

CHRISTINA: *A lot of people struggle to drink enough water—I know I used to. For me, the key is to make it easily accessible all day long. I keep a giant bottle of water with me at all times so I can chug some before I leave for work, while I'm on set, and again on my way home. I also make sure it's the only thing I'm drinking during the day.*

WHAT TO AVOID:

- All alcohol, caffeine, and tobacco. Feel free to replace your coffee with herbal tea or decaffeinated green, white, or rooibos teas. If you absolutely must have coffee, limit it to one cup a day.

CHRISTINA: *I know skipping your morning coffee seems like a nonstarter, but if I can do it, you can do it! By day two or three, I was surprised to find that I wasn't missing caffeine at all.*

- All dairy, gluten, refined sugar, and processed foods.

- Eat as many and as much of the Reset-approved foods as you want. It is very difficult to overeat the foods on this plan!
- Begin each day with lemon water. Just add a squeeze of fresh lemon juice to a glass of room-temperature or warm water and drink up.
- Eat your first meal within one hour of waking, then every three to four hours after that—no longer. The actual time you eat your meals is inconsequential as long as you are eating within the three-to-four-hour window.

CHRISTINA: *Having meals ready to go so you can grab them and go is crucial. You can prep most of the smoothies ahead of time by tossing the ingredients in a freezer-safe jar, storing them in the freezer, then simply dumping it all in a blender with some nut milk or coconut water. Done and done.*

- Eat intuitively: Use this time to learn your body's hunger and fullness cues. Eat until you are satisfied (but not stuffed). Pay close attention to how food affects your body and mind, as well as how you feel after each meal.

TIPS:

- Aim to drink two to three cups of tea per day, either herbal or decaffeinated green. Green tea is packed with health-promoting antioxidants, and some studies have found that it increases the body's ability to burn fat for energy.
- Keep healthy snacks like nuts and seeds as well as whole fruit on hand in case of "emergency" hunger attacks.
- Use homemade salad dressings whenever possible. If purchased, look for the shortest, cleanest ingredients list with no added sugar, MSG, or preservatives. You can also use a squeeze of lemon or splash of vinegar with a drizzle of high-quality extra-virgin olive oil for a quick, delicious dressing.

- Use healthy plant oils like olive, avocado, coconut, sunflower, and grapeseed oils for cooking or as a base for dressings.
- Enjoy seeds like chia, flax, and hemp hearts to get a dose of fiber, protein, and healthy omegas. They can be added to smoothies or sprinkled over oatmeal, salads, nut butters, and other dishes.
- Feel free to switch meals around or repeat meals that you like—and it's perfectly fine to eat leftovers for lunch the next day. As long as you're getting in your five colors a day, you're eating enough variety.

CHRISTINA: *Leftovers heaped on top of a bed of greens = best lunch or dinner ever. I'm also all for having smoothies for just about any meal of the day.*

THE 14-DAY RESET MEAL PLAN

WEEK 1

Day 1

UPON WAKING:

16 ounces room-temperature lemon water + probiotic

Drink 16 ounces water with each meal and sip additional water throughout the day.

BREAKFAST (7 AM)

Lemon-Ginger Detox Smoothie (page 184)

SNACK (10 AM)

Hearty Veggie Egg Cups (page 195): Enjoy 2 to 3 with salsa (no sugar added)

½ cup strawberries

LUNCH (1 PM)

Cucumber Ribbon Salad (page 226)

SNACK (4 PM)

Ruby grapefruit

¼ cup nuts of your choice (cashews, pistachios, almonds, walnuts, macadamias, or a mixture)

DINNER (7 PM)

Greek Potato Salad (page 227)

CHRISTINA'S TIP: *Make extra for lunch tomorrow!*

YOUR NEW MORNING RITUAL

You'll notice that we recommend starting your day with 16 ounces (2 cups) of water with lemon and a probiotic. There are a number of reasons why it's a good idea to kick things off with this combo: Your body loses hydration as it sleeps, so it's important to restore that water, especially as your digestion ramps up for the day. Adding lemon juice also

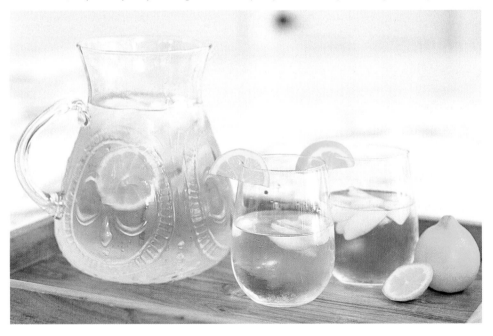

stimulates your digestive fire, while contributing enzymes that help break down food, as well as antioxidants and phytonutrients that support your body's natural defense mechanisms. By pairing this simple tonic with a probiotic supplement, you'll also be readying your gut for a day of receiving your food and ensuring that it is broken down and processed effectively. While the beneficial bacteria in your gut will get plenty of nourishment from all the whole-plant fiber you'll be eating during the Reset, taking a probiotic supplement is like an insurance policy that your gut flora stays as robust and diverse as possible. Because optimal gut health doesn't just require having healthy bacteria, it's also about having a wide array of strains. So when choosing a supplement, look for one that offers diversity in types of bacteria.

Day 2

UPON WAKING:

16 ounces room-temperature lemon water + probiotic

Drink 16 ounces water with each meal and sip additional water throughout the day.

BREAKFAST (7 AM)

Lemon-Ginger Detox Smoothie (page 184)

SNACK (10 AM)

2 to 3 leftover Hearty Veggie Egg Cups

½ grapefruit

LUNCH (1 PM)

2 cups spring salad mix topped with 1 serving leftover Greek Potato Salad

SNACK (4 PM)

Hummus Power Bowl (page 223)

DINNER (7 PM)

California Chicken Bowl (page 220)

Day 3

UPON WAKING:

16 ounces room-temperature lemon water + probiotic

Drink 16 ounces water with each meal and sip additional water throughout the day.

BREAKFAST (7 AM)

Lemon-Ginger Detox Smoothie (page 184)

SNACK (10 AM)

Baked Oatmeal Bars (page 207): Enjoy 3 to 4

1 hard-boiled egg

LUNCH (1 PM)

Strawberry Tossed Salad (page 225)

SNACK (4 PM)

Leftover Hummus Power Bowl

DINNER (7 PM)

Pineapple Stir-Fry (page 241)

CHRISTINA'S TIP: *Make PB&J Overnight Oats (page 199) for tomorrow's snack.*

Day 4

UPON WAKING:

16 ounces room-temperature lemon water + probiotic

Drink 16 ounces water with each meal and sip additional water throughout the day.

BREAKFAST (7 AM)

Cherry-Berry Pie Smoothie (page 186)

SNACK (10 AM)

PB&J Overnight Oats (page 199)

LUNCH (1 PM)

Taco Salad (page 230) served over 1 cup mixed shredded cabbage

SNACK (4 PM)

2 hard-boiled eggs

1 cup mixed berries (cherries, blueberries, blackberries, raspberries, strawberries, etc.)

DINNER (7 PM)

Salmon & Veggies (page 242)

CHRISTINA'S TIP: *You can make the Taco Salad the night before, but if you make the guacamole ahead of time, store it with the avocado pit and squeeze extra lime juice over the top to prevent browning.*

Day 5

UPON WAKING:

16 ounces room-temperature lemon water + probiotic
Drink 16 ounces water with each meal and sip additional water throughout the day.

BREAKFAST (7 AM)

Cherry-Berry Pie Smoothie (page 186)

SNACK (10 AM)

Choco Maca Chia Pudding (page 188)

CHRISTINA'S TIP: *Make extra for the family if you don't want them to eat all of yours!*

LUNCH (1 PM)

Fermented Cucumber Salad (page 224)

CHRISTINA'S TIP: *Why fermented veggies? Fermented foods boost healthy gut bacteria, which makes food easier to absorb, slows digestion, and optimizes the nutrients we are eating from superfoods.*

SNACK (4 PM)

2 rice cakes with ½ avocado, smashed, and sliced hard-boiled egg on top

DINNER (7 PM)

Loaded Veggie White Chili (page 248)

Day 6

UPON WAKING:

16 ounces room-temperature lemon water + probiotic
Drink 16 ounces water with each meal and sip additional water throughout the day.

BREAKFAST (7 AM)

Cinnamon-Pear Smoothie (page 185)

SNACK (10 AM)

2 eggs over-easy topped with ½ cup chicken sausage or canned beans
1 grapefruit

LUNCH (1 PM)

Leftover Fermented Cucumber Salad

SNACK (4 PM)

Baked sweet potato topped with ½ cup sliced strawberries, 2 tablespoons peanut
  or almond butter, and 1 teaspoon hemp seeds

DINNER (7 PM)

Kitchen Sink Salad (page 235)

CHRISTINA'S TIP: *Double the recipe and save enough for tomorrow's lunch!*

Day 7

UPON WAKING:

16 ounces room-temperature lemon water + probiotic

Drink 16 ounces water with each meal and sip additional water throughout the day.

BREAKFAST (7 AM)

Cinnamon-Pear Smoothie (page 185)

SNACK (10 AM)

2 hard-boiled eggs

¾ cup fruit salad (berries, kiwi, pear, nectarine, etc.)

LUNCH (1 PM)

Leftover Kitchen Sink Salad served over 1 cup chopped spinach

SNACK (4 PM)

Craving Crusher Granola (page 208)

DINNER (7 PM)

Chicken Zucchini Burgers (page 238)

    Serve with Roasted Veggies: chop sweet potato, onion, and Brussel sprouts; toss on a baking sheet with a drizzle of avocado oil, salt, and pepper to taste; and bake at 425°F for 25 minutes, until tender and slightly caramelized.

    or

Store-bought veggie burger—I like Hilary's brand

    or

Skip the burger and serve the roasted veggies over ½ cup wild rice or quinoa, topped with 1 tablespoon of hemp seeds

WEEK 1

Christina: When it comes to getting healthy food in the house, planning ahead is essential. That's why every time I get ready for a Reset, I make a shopping list. (I LOVE lists—they're a crucial part of my life and my favorite way to clear up a little space in my mind, zero in on what I have to get done, and, of course, get organized. If it's not on the list, it probably won't happen!)

The first time I did the Reset, the list looked huge—I needed to buy a wider variety of fruits, vegetables, and herbs (i.e., more colors) than ever before; plus foods like dates, honey, pistachios, and olives, which I once considered too indulgent but now know are essential for making Cara's signature smoothies and salads. I had to stock my dry goods stash with plenty of flax meal, oats, quinoa, and beans; fill my spice drawer with anti-inflammatory turmeric, blood sugar–stabilizing cinnamon, and mineralizing pink Himalayan salt; and take a leap of faith on new healing foods like fermented veggies, maca, and cacao. But once I started following Cara's approach to intuitive eating, my shopping lists got smaller and more manageable since I already had all the basics (which, except for fresh produce, last for a really long time if stored properly). Now I love looking through my pantry and peeking into my fridge and seeing all the delicious options I have for whipping up something to eat, and knowing that I always have something healthy to feed the kids.

The list that follows is a basic inventory of what you'll want to have on hand for your first week detoxing. Read it through and first cross off any items you already have in your kitchen—I bet you have a bunch! Next, decide who you're going to be preparing the meals for: just yourself, you and your partner, your family, etc. That way you'll know exactly how much to buy. And if there's a food that you're really not into, feel free to swap it out with another meal you prefer—we're going for maximum tastiness here. Most important, don't forget your list!

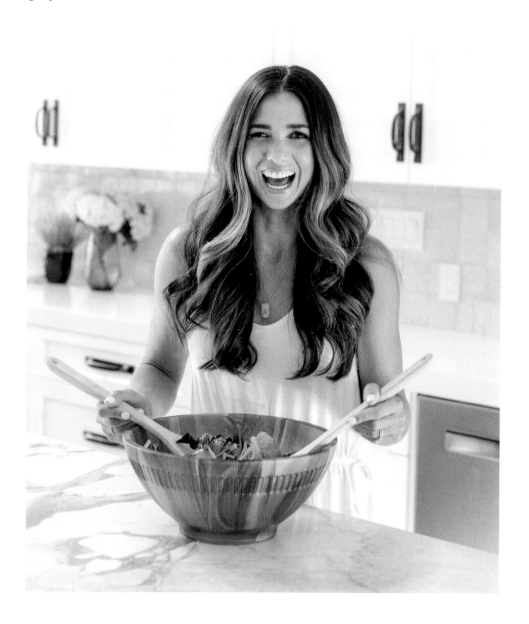

RESET SHOPPING LIST

FRUITS

apples (Granny Smith)

avocados

bananas

berries: strawberries, blueberries, raspberries, and blackberries

grapefruit

lemons

pears

pineapple

VEGETABLES AND HERBS

asparagus

basil

bell peppers: red, green, yellow, and orange → *Yellow and orange tend to be sweeter—perfect if you're a bell pepper skeptic. Kids also love the bright colors!*

Bibb or Boston lettuce

broccoli

Brussels sprouts

cabbage (green and purple)

carrots (shredded and baby)

cauliflower

celery

cilantro → *Did you know that cilantro helps the body detoxify while also keeping your blood sugar stable?*

corn

cucumber

dill

garlic

ginger root/ginger paste

green beans

green onions

green peas (frozen are okay)

jicama → *Super-hydrating, crunchy, and mildly flavored—perfect for the kiddos to munch and dip, too.*

kale

mint → *Awesome if you need a little help in the digestion department.*

mixed spring greens

onion: Vidalia, brown, red, and yellow

parsley

red potatoes

rhubarb (fresh or frozen, substitute celery if unavailable)

romaine lettuce

shallots

spinach

sweet potatoes

tomatoes (cherry or grape and Roma)

PROTEINS

beans: organic black beans

boneless, skinless chicken breasts

chicken sausage

eggs

hummus → *Keep it clean with a few ingredients you recognize and no soybean oil.*

lean ground turkey breast (or grass-fed bison)

nuts and seeds: pepitas, walnuts, cashews, almonds, pistachios, pine nuts, sesame seeds

nut/seed butters: almond, natural peanut, cashew → *Substitute sunflower seed butter or tahini if you're allergic to nuts or just want to change it up!*

salmon fillets (wild-caught)

seeds: hemp, chia, sunflower

shrimp (wild)

DRY GOODS

brown rice or wild rice cakes

cacao powder → *So chocolatey, so good! And it helps control blood sugar, blood pressure, and inflammation.*

flax meal/ground flax seeds

gluten-free pasta (brown rice and quinoa pasta)

maca root powder → *One of my favorite superfoods because it gently boosts energy, balances hormones, and reduces anxiety. Plus it has a malty sweet taste.*

nutritional yeast

pitted dates

quinoa

rolled oats

unsweetened dried fruit

unsweetened shredded coconut

wild or brown rice

REFRIGERATED AND FROZEN

bag of riced cauliflower

frozen mango

OILS AND SPICES

black pepper

cinnamon

ground ginger

oils (avocado and extra-virgin olive)

pink Himalayan sea salt

pumpkin pie spice

red pepper flakes or cayenne pepper

turmeric

PANTRY ITEMS

apple cider vinegar

artichoke hearts

canned coconut cream→ *Did you ever think a nutritionist would make you buy something so tasty?! This is smoothie gold.*

capers

coconut aminos → *Same salty zing as soy sauce but without the soy.*

coconut mayo (Primal Kitchen or Chosen Foods brands)

Dijon mustard

Kalamata olives

low-sodium Worcestershire sauce

pickles or other fermented vegetables → *Gives your gut a boost of healthy bacteria!*

pure maple syrup

pure vanilla extract

raw honey → *Should say "raw" on the label, meaning it hasn't been heated and still has all of its good-for-you enzymes and antioxidants.*

rice vinegar

salsa → *Make sure there are no additives; freshly made is best.*

sauerkraut

unsweetened coconut water or nut milk

veggie and/or chicken bone broth

WEEK 1

Christina: As you finish up the first week of the Reset, take a moment to thank yourself for giving your body such an incredible gift. This isn't easy! It's one thing to make a big shift in your daily habits, it's quite another to do it while you're dealing with everything else that life throws your way. So before you move on to Week 2, check in with yourself. How's your body feeling? Any differences between Day 1 and Day 7? I highly recommend writing down anything that comes to mind. That way, if in a week or a month you feel like you aren't making progress or you find yourself losing your way down the road, you can look back at these notes to reassure yourself that you can create positive shifts in your body and mind, and that you have the blueprint for doing just that. Not everything you've experienced will have been positive—that's okay! Those experiences are just as valid, namely as reminders that your body had to do a lot of work to shift from old patterns. That's why we wanted to take this opportunity to give you the tools to continue to make that shift, specifically regarding how you talk to yourself.

Mini Mind-set Challenge

We'll get into more detail about the importance of mindfulness in chapter 7, but because it's such an essential part of healing—and because we're hitting the Reset button—Cara and I wanted to start the shift now. Many of us get in the habit of rushing from place to place and have an inner dialogue that runs on autopilot. For me, driving the busy L.A. freeways every morning can be frustrating, and I often find myself thinking critical thoughts about the other drivers around me. This kind of mind-set is not particularly useful and leaves me feeling anxious and stressed in the morning. But when I take a moment to practice compassion and understanding toward myself and others, I start to notice the beautiful world around me—the mountains, the ocean, a family member or friend I want to pray for, or just the great song playing on the radio.

Cara: Practicing mindfulness starts with observing your thoughts without judgment. Are you critical of your health goals, your body, or your parenting? Are you judgmental of your partner, children, or other parents? Maybe you're frustrated after waiting a long time at the doctor's office, or in the carpool line at school, or perhaps someone is late meeting you. As the thoughts come up, notice them but try not to react to them emotionally.

Then, reframe your inner dialogue by asking, "How would I react if it were my best friend saying these things to me?" Imagine if she said one of the many things you'd said to yourself about herself, something like, "I can't believe I skipped my workout again today. I'm so lazy." What do you think you'd say to her? That she's right? No way! You'd say, "Listen, you're doing the best you can and you're juggling a lot right now. You are not lazy—and tomorrow is a new day!" So why not offer yourself the same compassion? This also goes for the thoughts you have about other people. Recognize that you don't always know their story and what they might be struggling with that day. Try leading with the same compassion you're going to start showing yourself. For example, "If her life is anything like mine, then there's probably a good reason why she's running late; I'm just grateful I was able to make it on time." To help you practice this compassionate reframing, I've included a worksheet that I give all my clients.

Inner Dialogue and Self-Talk Worksheet

Example 1:

SELF-STATEMENT: I'm so lazy! Why can't I just work out and do my meal prep when I get up in the morning? This is too hard.

REFRAME: Change is hard, but I've got this. It's just daily improvements. I can substitute a good, healthy meal even though I didn't meal prep, and I'll walk at lunch and take the stairs. There's always a solution.

Example 2:

INNER DIALOGUE: I can't believe that mom I met at the playground lets her kids get away with such terrible behavior. It's so rude! Why can't she control her kids?

REFRAME: She must be going through a lot. Parenting is tough! I wonder if she has any help or support. I'm so grateful for the support I have.

Your turn!

Current Self-Statement/Belief: _____

_____

Reframe: _____

_____

Current Self-Statement/Belief: _____

_____

Reframe: _____

_____

THE 14-DAY RESET MEAL PLAN

Day 8

UPON WAKING:

16 ounces room-temperature lemon water + probiotic

Drink 16 ounces water with each meal and sip additional water throughout the day.

BREAKFAST (7 AM)

Green Mango Blast Smoothie (page 187)

SNACK (10 AM)

2 brown rice cakes topped with:

2 hard-boiled eggs, sliced or chopped, seasoned with black pepper

¼ avocado, smashed, sprinkled with hemp seeds and red pepper flakes or
    cayenne pepper

LUNCH (1 PM)

Leftover Chicken Zucchini Burgers or store-bought veggie burger

Serve over a bed of romaine lettuce or mixed greens with ¼ cup shredded carrots, 5 to 6 cherry tomatoes, sauerkraut, ¼ avocado, and dressing of choice.

SNACK (4 PM)

2 Harvest Oat Muffins (page 203)

DINNER (7 PM)

Satay Lettuce Wraps (page 257)

CHRISTINA'S TIP: *Store leftover Satay Lettuce Wraps filling to enjoy over greens tomorrow.*

Day 9

UPON WAKING:

16 ounces room-temperature lemon water + probiotic

Drink 16 ounces water with each meal and sip additional water throughout the day.

BREAKFAST (7 AM)

Green Mango Blast Smoothie (page 187)

SNACK (10 AM)

2 hard-boiled eggs

½ cup grapes

½ cup berries

LUNCH (1 PM)

Leftover Satay Lettuce Wraps filling over 2 cups of greens

SNACK (4 PM)

Unlimited raw colorful non-starchy veggies (bell peppers, broccoli, celery, cucumber, cauliflower, jicama, sugar snap peas, *or* cherry/grape tomatoes)

¼ cup hummus

DINNER (7 PM)

Taco Tuesday! Coconut Shrimp Tacos with Mango Salsa and Avocado Cilantro Sauce (page 245)

Day 10

UPON WAKING:

16 ounces room-temperature lemon water + probiotic

Drink 16 ounces water with each meal and sip additional water throughout the day.

BREAKFAST (7 AM)

Green Mango Blast Smoothie (page 187)

SNACK (10 AM)

Craving Crusher Granola (page 208)

LUNCH (1 PM)

Crunchy Coleslaw (page 229)

SNACK (4 PM)

1 cup herbal/rooibos/white/green tea, served hot or iced—however you like it!

1 medium apple

2 tablespoons natural nut/seed butter (or Justin's nut butter packet)

Sprinkle of cinnamon and hemp seeds

DINNER (7 PM)

BBQ Chicken-Stuffed Peppers (page 260)

CHRISTINA'S TIP: *Those dinner leftovers become lunch tomorrow—pack them up to eat over a bed of greens.*

Day 11

BEGIN TO TRANSITION DAIRY BACK IN

Pay close attention to how you feel as you add dairy back into your diet. Be mindful of side effects (if any), including changes in digestion, bathroom habits, skin and hair, energy level, mental clarity/focus, head or body aches, irritability, or food cravings. Make notes in your food log accordingly.

UPON WAKING:

16 ounces room-temperature lemon water + probiotic

Drink 16 ounces water with each meal and sip additional water throughout the day.

BREAKFAST (7 AM)

Banana-Vanilla-Fig Smoothie (page 183)

SNACK (10 AM)

Scramble 2 eggs and mix with all the veggies you want. Enjoy with fresh fruit.

LUNCH (1 PM)

Leftover BBQ Chicken-Stuffed Peppers over 2 cups of greens

SNACK (4 PM)

Homemade Vanilla-Cinnamon Pecan Butter (page 267)

1 cup fresh fruit of your choice, cut up for dipping (choose multiple colors if possible!)

DINNER (7 PM)

4 to 6 ounces grilled wild white fish (cod, grouper, sole, etc.), seasoned simply with fresh herbs, lemon zest, fresh lemon juice, salt, and pepper

½ cup steamed or roasted baby carrots, seasoned with salt and pepper

½ cup cooked brown or wild rice, cooked in bone broth for added flavor and nutrients

Serve with Cucumber Ribbon Salad (page 226)

CHRISTINA'S TIP: *Make PB&J Overnight Oats (page 199) for tomorrow's snack.*

Day 12

UPON WAKING:

16 ounces room-temperature lemon water + probiotic

Drink 16 ounces water with each meal and sip additional water throughout the day.

BREAKFAST (7 AM)

Banana-Vanilla-Fig Smoothie (page 183)

SNACK (10 AM)

PB&J Overnight Oats (page 199)

LUNCH (1 PM)

Mexican Caesar Salad (page 233)

SNACK (4 PM)

2 full-fat string cheese sticks

1 kiwi

½ cup berries

DINNER (7 PM)

Chicken Tortilla Soup (page 251)

CHRISTINA'S TIP: *Make a batch of Coconut-Pistachio Chia Pudding (page 188) to have for breakfast tomorrow and on Day 14.*

Day 13

BEGIN TO TRANSITION GLUTEN BACK IN

Pay close attention to how you feel as you add gluten back into your diet. Be mindful of side effects (if any), including changes in digestion, bathroom habits, skin and hair, energy level, mental clarity/focus, head or body aches, irritability, or food cravings. Make notes in your food log accordingly.

UPON WAKING:

16 ounces room-temperature lemon water + probiotic

Drink 16 ounces water with each meal and sip additional water throughout the day.

BREAKFAST (7 AM)

Coconut-Pistachio Chia Pudding (page 188)

SNACK (10 AM)

1 slice sprouted whole grain (or gluten-free) toast topped with:

¼ cup cottage cheese

¼ avocado

Tomato slices sprinkled with salt, pepper, and hemp seeds

LUNCH (1 PM)

Leftover Chicken Tortilla Soup with Cucumber Ribbon Salad (page 226)

SNACK (4 PM)

2 brown or wild rice cakes topped with:

2 tablespoons unsweetened nut/seed butter and a sprinkle of hemp seeds

½ cup berries

DINNER (7 PM)

Quick Cannellini & Spinach Pasta (page 243)

Day 14

UPON WAKING:

16 ounces room-temperature lemon water + probiotic

Drink 16 ounces water with each meal and sip additional water throughout the day.

BREAKFAST (7 AM)

Coconut-Pistachio Chia Pudding (page 188)

SNACK (10 AM)

Pumpkin-Pecan Pancakes (page 192)

CHRISTINA'S TIP: *Double or even triple the recipe and save extras in the fridge or freezer for quick meals throughout the week!*

LUNCH (1 PM)

Leftover Quick Cannellini & Spinach Pasta

SNACK (4 PM)

2 full-fat string cheese sticks

1 cup grapes

DINNER (7 PM)

Campfire Packets (page 258)

WEEK 2

HIT THE STORE

Christina: I'm back with more lists! By now you know the drill: Cross off what you have left over from Week 1 and think about which of these meals you can get more mileage out of by either doubling up so you have leftovers or making a family meal out of them. This list will look very similar to last week's, namely because each of the recommended recipes calls for a similar rotation of fresh, healing foods. So maybe this week you can take a chance and try a new ingredient that you weren't so sure about last week!

RESET SHOPPING LIST

FRUITS

apples

avocados

bananas

berries: blackberries,
strawberries, blueberries,
and raspberries

grapes

kiwi

lemons

limes

mangos → *Pro tip: If you're too intimidated to peel and pit fresh mangos, buy frozen.*

oranges

pineapple

plantains → *These cook up just like potatoes but have more vitamins, minerals, and fiber*

VEGETABLES AND HERBS

bell peppers: red, green,
yellow, orange

broccoli → *Don't underestimate how yummy broccoli can be—when you cook it right and give it lots of flavor with fresh herbs and spices, it's a game-changer.*

cabbage (red)

carrots (large and/or baby)

cauliflower

celery

cilantro

corn

cucumbers (baby and/or
regular)

dill

garlic

green onions

jicama

mint

mixed greens

mushrooms

onions (Vidalia and red)

oregano

parsley

radishes → *These add spicy crunch to just about everything, and they have a ton of water content.*

romaine lettuce

shallots

spaghetti squash → *The insides cook up just like noodles and are perfect for tossing with lots of sauce.*

spinach

sugar snap peas

tomatoes (cherry or grape
and Roma) → *We eat small tomatoes like candy in our house!*

zucchini

PROTEINS

beans: black, cannellini,
pinto

chicken sausage

eggs

hummus (clean with short
ingredient list)

lentils

nut/seed butters: almond,
natural peanut → *Note: You can substitute sunflower seed butter.*

nuts: almonds, cashews,
walnuts

nitrate-free turkey breast

seeds: chia, hemp

salmon fillets (wild-caught)

shrimp (wild)

skinless chicken
tenderloins

wild white fish (code, sole,
grouper)

DRY GOODS

brown rice or wild rice cakes → *The perfect vehicle to get more nut butter or smashed avocado into your mouth*

cacao powder

corn tortillas

dark chocolate chips → *I'm always SO excited to see these back on the list!*

flax meal/ground flax seeds

maca root power

nutritional yeast → *A pantry secret weapon— it has a nutty, cheesy flavor, and you can sprinkle it on just about anything, from pasta to popcorn.*

pitted dates

quinoa

rolled oats

unsweetened dried fruit

whole grain or gluten-free pasta

whole grain sprouted bread

wild or brown rice

REFRIGERATED AND FROZEN

bag of cauliflower rice

cottage cheese

frozen fruit: cherries, mangos, mixed berries

frozen peas

grass-fed butter or ghee

Parmesan cheese

pico de gallo or fresh salsa

plain Greek yogurt (2 percent)

string cheese sticks (full-fat)

OILS AND SPICES

black pepper

cardamom → *Little-known fact: In addition to having a sweet flavor, cardamom is a natural anti-inflammatory, antioxidant, diuretic, and digestion-soother.*

cayenne

chili powder

cinnamon

cumin

oils: avocado, coconut, extra-virgin olive, sesame

oregano

paprika

pink Himalayan sea salt

red pepper flakes

PANTRY ITEMS

artichoke hearts

baking soda

black olives

chicken bone broth (low-sodium)

coconut aminos

coconut milk (full-fat)

crushed tomatoes

diced green chilies

fermented veggies: kimchi and/or sauerkraut → *Now's your chance to get adventurous! I love spicy kimchi, especially chopped up in salads.*

peppermint extract

pure maple syrup

pure vanilla extract

raw honey

unsweetened coconut beverage or nut milk

vinegars: apple cider, balsamic, red wine

Back to Everyday Life

Cara: With the detox behind you, you should be feeling revitalized, clear-headed, and lighter in body, mind, and spirit. You have a working idea of the foods that may not be contributing to your overall wellness, as well as firsthand proof that eating for stable blood sugar, getting in a wide variety of fruits and vegetables, and combining your macronutrients contribute to your feeling like you could take on the world. So now the question is: How do you keep the momentum going post-Reset?

Luckily, you've already mastered the fundamentals of intuitive eating during the detox, and you've tackled the really difficult part: planning ahead. Planning is everything when it comes to maintaining a health-promoting diet that doesn't feel restrictive or overwhelming. That doesn't mean having to map out every piece of food that goes into your mouth—that would be impossible! What I mean is being able to set yourself up for success by doing the heavy lifting ahead of time. That includes:

- Making sure your pantry and fridge are stocked with foods that you love and that you know you can use to assemble quick meals and snacks.
- Prepping ingredients in advance: Wash and chop your veggies so they're ready for dipping, tossing, or sautéing; cook big batches of beans or grains; set up some overnight oats; whip up a couple dressings; make healthy meals too easy *not* to make.

Thinking a few steps ahead is particularly important if you're busy—which I'm guessing includes about 99 percent of you! By having ingredients ready for the grabbing, assembling, or cooking, all you have to do is check in with yourself and think, *What do I feel like eating?* And for the days when the going

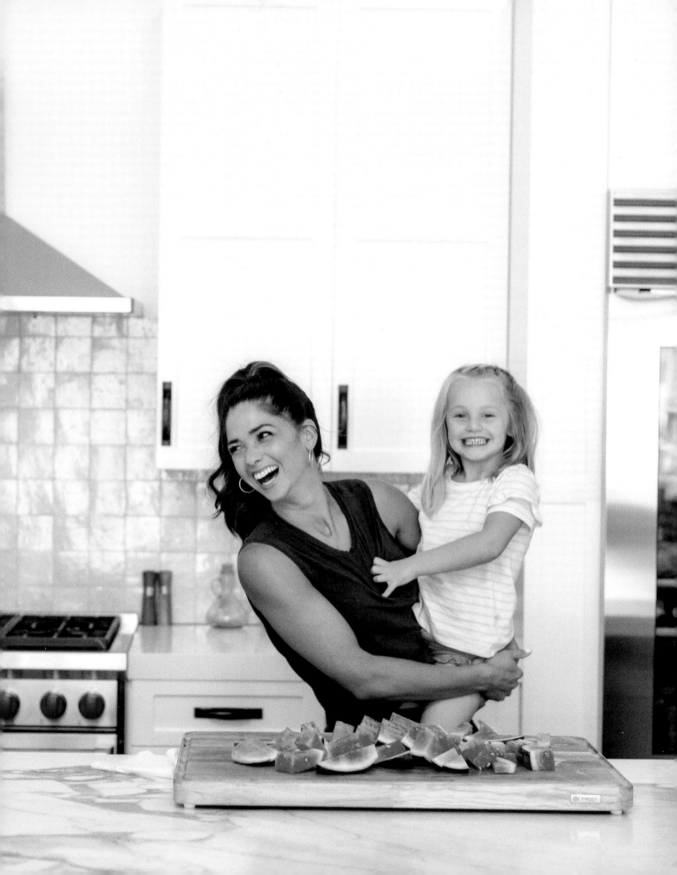

really gets tough, you don't even have think! Christina has become a pro when it comes to figuring out which ingredients are going to get her the most mileage with mix-and-match meals and snacks. Check out chapter 8 for the tips and hacks that we rely on to get us through this craziness we call life!

Maintenance and Troubleshooting

It's happened to all of us: You're going along, feeling great, but every now and then you take some . . . liberties. Maybe you're traveling, hitting the holiday party circuit, or having one of those weeks (months?) when regular grocery shopping and meal prepping just isn't in the cards. Don't worry! It's completely normal. The best part about intuitive eating is that it's not all-or-nothing. Every day is a fresh new day—heck, every meal is a fresh new opportunity to give your body what it needs to feel great and serve you well.

I also recommend detoxing regularly. Hitting the reset button on your metabolism is a rhythm as natural as the seasons. That's why I suggest that my clients undergo a 14-Day Reset four times a year, during the transition between each season. It's not only a way to reinvigorate your body and each of its systems (immune, digestive, endocrine, neurological), it's also an opportunity to reflect on how you're feeling. Are there any symptoms that you've started to accept as "normal," like daily headaches, skin conditions, bloating, or irregular digestion? Do you feel rested in the morning, or are you still exhausted—no matter how much sleep you've gotten? Do rigorous workouts leave you down for the count for a few days? Are you catching every bug that your kids bring home from school? If you're not feeling your best, then there's a chance that there are still foods in your diet that aren't supporting your health. These aren't necessarily the usual culprits—dairy, gluten, and processed sugar. As Christina discovered, eating too many nuts and nut butters was holding her back from feeling her best, so she cut back to having them a couple times a week instead of every day. Every body is different, which is why there's no one-size-fits-all solution, and why you ultimately have to be your own detective. You'll want to keep notes of how you feel after each meal and see if you can connect the dots between the ingredients in your meals and snacks and your symptoms. The more you tune in and listen, the more success you'll have down the road when it comes to making choices that support your health.

Christina: If you're still not feeling great after your Reset, you may want to consider consulting an integrative doctor. Unlike traditional medical doctors, who tend to diagnose and treat individual symptoms instead of doing a complete evaluation that takes into account all of your bodily systems, integrative doctors make it their goal to assess your body, lifestyle, mind, and spirit as one package deal. They'll typically take one to two hours during your intake, asking you interview-style questions about everything from what you eat, to how much stress you have, to how much you poop (a major insight into your health!). They'll also run much more detailed blood work than a general practitioner in order to get a clearer sense of what may be going on in your body. Starting in my thirties when my autoimmune symptoms really began to creep up, I consulted integrative doctors because I wanted to know why these things were happening in my body and how I could actively make them better—without just popping a pill. Although integrative doctors can and will give you medication, it's typically in addition to other lifestyle changes that will help in the long run, like making better nutritional choices, reducing stress, getting bodywork treatments such as Reiki or acupuncture, or practicing yoga. Seeing an integrative practitioner can be expensive and is not always covered by insurance, but the insight you get from one visit will go a long way. Even an annual tune-up will do the trick!

The 80/20 Rule, aka Nobody's Perfect
(nor should they be)

Cara: While there's no denying that the other five guidelines are the best way to help you reach optimal physical health, this one is crucial for your emotional health, especially as you're easing into this new approach to eating. I want you to hear this: There is no such thing as "perfect" eating or a "perfect" day. Both Christina and I love our desserts, cocktails, and other special treats. We go out to dinner with our husbands; we enjoy a ladies' night out with our friends; and we're all-around human. So when it comes time to apply these guidelines to your life, I recommend doing so with balance, positive self-talk, and clear intentions. Here are my tips for doing just that:

1. STOP ASSIGNING MORALITY TO FOOD/LIFESTYLE CHOICES. What you eat is not "right" or "wrong," nor does eating something indulgent make you a "bad" person.

2. BREAK NEGATIVE THINKING PATTERNS. For many people, negative patterns related to their eating habits looks something like this:

    Bad meal → bad day → bad week → bad month . . . etc.

Replace negative thinking patterns with new positive affirmations. For example:

- I am who I am and I like who I am!
- Today is a new day and a new beginning, a chance to be whomever I want to be.
- I let go of old limitations. I am at peace with myself. I am motivated!
- I am in the process of making positive changes in all areas of my life, and I am committed to the time it takes to make those changes.

3. **DON'T RESTRICT YOURSELF.** Restrictive mind-sets or labeling certain foods as "off-limits" only makes your brain focus on these things and crave them more intensely. Instead of all or nothing, use 80/20 as a loose guideline—as in, truly enjoying (with zero guilt!) the foods you love that might not be the best for you about 20 percent of the time. Over time, you won't feel like you need to monitor this closely because you'll know when you've been overdoing it with foods that don't serve your health.

4. **BE INTENTIONAL.** When we go out for date night or get together with friends, our intention is to celebrate and connect with the people we love. That means a glass of Prosecco, a bowl of freshly made pasta, an amazing dessert—whatever sounds nourishing to the *spirit*. But pro tip: If you're going out for drinks, avoid the carb-y snacks and order some protein—it'll help with the hangover. Christina is notorious for asking for a side of shredded chicken with her margarita and chips!

5. **BE GENTLE WITH YOURSELF!** No one is asking you to be perfect. The important thing is that you're changing your relationship with food in a healthy way that will benefit your whole life.

Small Changes Make a Big Difference

Remember that every little change you make will lead to significant and long-lasting results. When followed as a set, these guidelines will take you to amazing new places, but that doesn't mean that you won't see results if you have a few slip-ups. Maybe you can just manage eating five colors a couple of times a week or you're eating every four hours but aren't getting all the "right" foods—that's okay! Every day, you will get one step closer to achieving your goals.

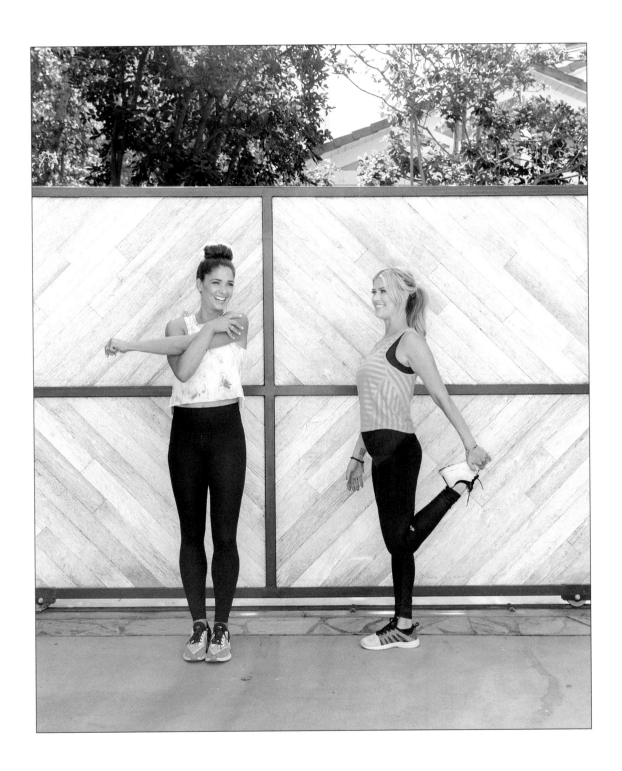

Part II

BUILDING
A STRONG
FOUNDATION

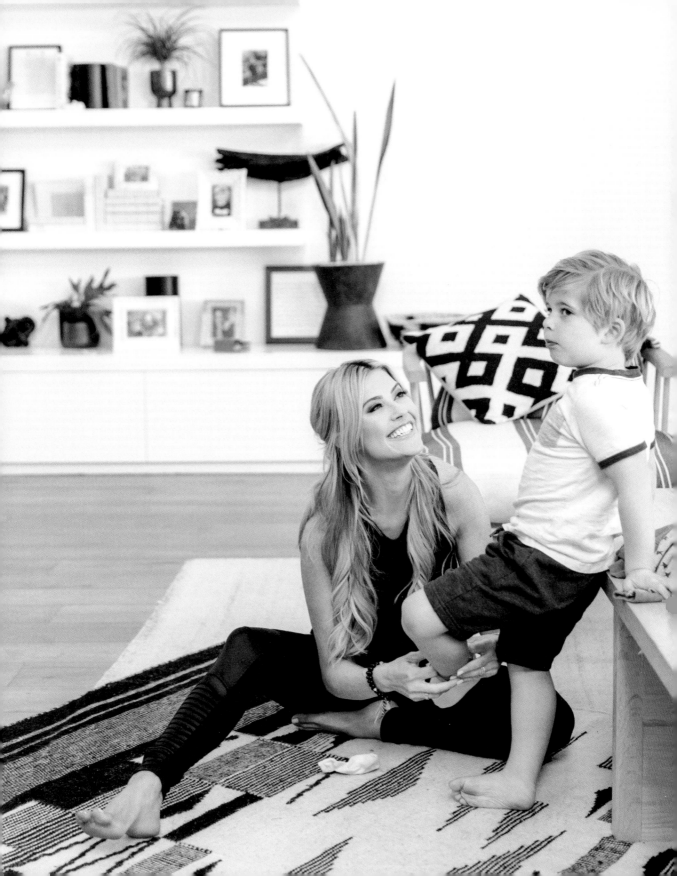

Chapter 4

PROJECT IN MOTION

Christina: I used to work out seven days a week, full on. We're talking dripping sweat. I've been an athlete from the time I was little and ran track in high school, so I've always felt my best when I get to move every day. But a few years ago, I started taking it to an extreme because I believed working out hard was what I "should" be doing, especially if I wanted to look good on TV. Then around the time I was having trouble getting pregnant with Brayden, I noticed that I wasn't recovering from exercise like I used to. In the past, working out always gave me energy, but I was finding that a tough workout could knock me on my butt for a week. My stomach would hurt, and I'd have zero stamina. I was learning the hard way that I needed to slow down, but I was worried that slowing down would mean gaining weight.

That's when Cara stepped in and helped me see that dialing things back was not a bad thing for my health or my weight. She taught me that not pushing my body so hard could rebalance my hormones and reduce the inflammation that was making my autoimmune symptoms worse. And she promised that working out smarter, not harder, would be the key to actually burning *more* fat. So I started scaling back, working out three or four days a week. I went for shorter, less intense runs, and I discovered the amazingness that is walking. Seriously, a good, brisk walk for thirty minutes is a magical thing. (And just about EVERYBODY can manage a walk every day!) I'd still go to the occasional Orangetheory or HIIT (high-intensity interval training) class if I was in the mood for a good sweat, but I listened to my body and made sure I wasn't overdoing it or going for longer than thirty to sixty minutes.

I also started doing yoga, which I NEVER thought I'd do because I'd always dismissed it as being either boring, annoying, or way too intense. But Cara's instructor showed me that when you have the right person guiding you, yoga is incredible. It made me feel strong *and* relaxed, a balance that I can adjust each day depending on how I'm feeling. I truly believe that everyone should be doing yoga, even if it's a super-simple, fifteen-to-twenty-minute session that you do before bed to wind down. We'll talk more about this in chapter 8, but you can find great videos online and pick one based on what you feel like your body needs that day.

Since I started scaling back, I have felt *way* better. I still get the benefits of exercise—mental and physical—and even though I'm working out way less often and with less intensely, I still wear the same size clothes. All I had to do was stop stressing out my body, start listening to what it needed, and then give it lots of variety to play with.

Cara: While food and nutrition are at the core of this program, exercise is crucial for living a balanced life. Christina and I both turn to exercise as a way to recharge and refresh, whether we're craving an all-out, high-intensity sweat session climbing stairs, running, or interval training; or something more restorative like walking, yoga, or body-weight exercises. We also believe that working out is about way more than just flat abs—it's about reducing stress, clearing your mind, and feeling more connected and creative.

We've dedicated this chapter to sharing the lessons that Christina and I have learned as we've changed our relationship with exercise: You don't need to work out for hours at a time every day to see great results; your body knows best when it comes to choosing what type of exercise to do; and exercise isn't just about physical transformation. You can absolutely achieve the results you want without wearing down your body and all of its systems. Because when we have a lot going on in our lives or maybe we haven't slept enough, exercise can actually put more stress on the body, which leads you right back to feeling not so great. The key is learning how to listen to what the body needs and wants. My hope for you is that you can tune in to this voice, understand the importance of exercise for your body *and* your brain, heal a negative relationship with exercise, and create a strong emotional connection with movement that you love.

Give Yourself Permission to Slow Down

There was a time in my life when, like Christina, I was working out six or seven days a week and at a very high intensity. It wasn't about punishment—it was fun! But, also like Christina, I wouldn't feel good afterward. I'd get nauseous, achy, and fatigued—like I couldn't get my blood sugar to stabilize.

And then I started getting injured, which had never happened before. But I pushed through—maybe because I felt like I had something to prove, because I was trying to outrun my anxiety, or because I wasn't feeling grounded and connected with others in my life (or myself). Regardless, my workouts had gone from being my biggest stress relief to causing more stress.

So I chilled the eff out. I started walking instead of running or climbing hundreds of stairs; I swapped high-intensity interval training for gentler, more controlled activities like Pilates, barre classes, and yoga. I counted running around with my kids or just doing some squats and planks while I cleaned up toys as exercise. And I gave myself permission not to work out for more than thirty minutes on most days. Not only did I see the same, if not better, results as far as feeling strong and lean, but I also felt like I was getting that amazing post-workout clarity back. Instead of pounding through hard-core workouts (which do have their own benefits and still pop up in my routine when I'm in the mood for a challenge) and tuning out to stay ahead of the burn, I was tuning *in*. I found my breath again, and that connected me even more deeply with my body.

That's when I reexamined everything I knew about exercise and came up with these new guidelines for an optimal movement practice:

- 30 minutes a session
- 4 times a week
- Maintaining a heart right of (220 minus your age) x .6 to .8

That's it. Just like my food program optimizes fat burning, so does this approach. If you maintain a heart rate in this range (and you'll be very surprised at how attainable and semi-comfortable that is), then you'll be much more efficient at accessing fat as your fuel source—without spending hours at the gym. Alternatively, when you stay in a high heart-rate zone (higher than

I've recommended) for an extended period of time (for most people, more than thirty minutes), you start burning muscle and depleting glycogen, an energy source that you store in your muscles. You also cause more significant wear and tear in your muscles and joints, which can lead to inflammation, and in turn, symptoms ranging from headaches and nausea to more serious chronic conditions.

It's also important to consider that the simple math equation we've always been taught—calories in minus calories burned = weight loss—isn't the whole picture. Yes, working out burns calories, but there are a lot of other variables that influence the function of your metabolism, including your sleep, your stress levels, and the quality of the food you eat. Exercise is an important part of a healthy lifestyle, but you don't need to over-exercise and under-eat to lose weight. You need to take better care of yourself!

AGE IS JUST A (HEART-RATE) NUMBER

Many of my clients who are obsessed with the idea that they should keep up the same level of fitness routine as they did in their twenties either wind up injured or chasing something that's just not going to make their bodies or their minds feel good. That's when they end up getting frustrated, throwing in the towel, and doing nothing. The better alternative—for you, your body, and your goals—is to stick with a heart rate that's unique to you and your body's physiological needs. And that means taking age into account!

When I used to train clients, they were always shocked when I would tell them to take a minute to breathe while their heart rate came down into the recommended range. That's because that range is the ideal zone for fat burning. This can include small spurts of high heart-rate intensity (like during a HIIT workout), but in order to stay in your fat-burning zone (and not your carb- or muscle-burning zone) you'll want to keep finding your way back to your target heart rate. When your heart rate is in the fat-burning zone, you don't have to spend hours at the gym to see results. And if you're not yet in the habit of regularly working out, don't feel like you need to ramp up the intensity right away. Go for a walk instead! Or find something else that makes you happy, whether that's swimming, boxing, dancing, or power walking. When I have clients who say they hate exercising, I tell them, "Then you're doing the wrong kind of exercise." There's something for everyone—you just gotta find your jam.

USE A HEART-RATE MONITOR

When we're starting a new routine, it's easy to focus on what we're not getting right—*I didn't sleep enough*; *I didn't eat well enough*; *I didn't exercise enough*. But oftentimes you're doing better than you think. That's why using a heart-rate monitor can be helpful, at least initially, until you get used to where your heart rate should ideally be during exercise (including non-exercise exercise, like walking the dog or playing with your kids). It's nice reassurance that, yes, you're doing a great job! My favorite monitor is the Fitbit Charge 3 because it's super accurate and light, but there are a variety of options out there. Choose one that works best for you.

Intuitive Movement

Christina: If you're anything like I was before I started working with Cara, then you might be skeptical of the idea that exercising *less* actually works. But the thing is, we are proof that it does! Cara and I—and hundreds of Cara's clients—are testimony to the fact that you can be kind to yourself and still look and feel your best. Granted, learning how to be gentle with myself and changing up my workouts depending on how I'm feeling has probably been the hardest lesson I've had to learn on this journey. But over time, it's gotten easier. If I have thirty minutes and I want to get in a good, sweaty workout, I'll go for a run (maybe with some walking breaks, if things get too intense). If I want something more hard-core, it's Orangetheory (though I always warn the instructor that he'd better not yell at me!). If I want to tone up but keep things less sweaty, I'll go to a barre class (it finally gave me a butt!). But if I feel like I'm getting sick or I haven't been sleeping well, then I'll cancel my workouts and go for a walk. And I don't get in my head about how many high-intensity workouts I get in a week because the most important thing to me is feeling good—and if something doesn't make me feel good, it's gotta go. The truth is, if you're eating for stable blood sugar, you're going to continue to burn fat, regardless of whether or not you work out. So I don't exercise to lose weight or look a certain way; I do it to keep my insides healthy, my mind sharp, my stress at bay, my heart joyful, and my creativity revved up.

Cara: In addition to the fact that your body doesn't need more exercise than outlined in my recommendations (30 minutes, 4 times a week), there's another reason why I keep this guideline minimal: because I know that once a client finds a way of moving that's pleasurable and not punishing, she's going to do more of it. It's a win-win: she gets to feel like an overachiever while also having the mental safety net of knowing that if things get busy (and they always get busy) and she has to scale back, she won't become derailed from her goals. Okay, I know I just totally blew my secret, but the moral of the story here is that our workouts should evolve and cycle as we evolve and cycle. And no program can tell you how your body should or shouldn't be feeling on a given day or month—only you can. A recent study published in the *Journal of Athletic Training* showed that a female athlete's risk of an ACL injury is greater just before she ovulates than after she ovulates. That's no coincidence! As our hormones shift, so does the strength and flexibility of our muscles, joints, and ligaments. Similarly, when we're sick, run-down, and stressed out, our bodies have bigger battles to fight than dealing with the inflammation caused by too-aggressive exercise. So if your body is politely asking for a slower pace, please honor that request. You'll be giving it a much more nourishing, healing boost by moving gently. Then, when you're back to feeling strong and invigorated, get that sweat on!

I think it's helpful to lead your fitness practice with gratitude, as well—gratitude that your body can get you out of bed in the morning and give you the ability to do the things you love; that your heart pumps healthy blood to keep your body strong; that getting yourself moving just a few times a week is enough to give you the gift of a stronger immune system by flushing bacteria out of your lungs and helping to generate more disease-fighting antibodies; for more even-keeled hormones and blood sugar owing to a balancing effect in the thyroid, adrenals, and pituitary glands; for an elevated mood thanks to nature's antianxiety medicine, endorphins; and for a clearer mind. To me, that beats looking good in a bathing suit any day.

Loving the
Body You Have

When I was in my twenties, I was caught in a bad cycle of disordered eating. I was laser-focused on attaining the "perfect body" and would restrict my eating and work out like crazy. It didn't help that I played basketball in college, and as an athlete I was hyper-competitive and very goal-oriented. I would set a goal for my body, achieve it, and then reset my goal—usually to get my size smaller or my weight even lower. At my unhealthiest point, I was a size 0, and such an unnatural size 0 that I felt uncomfortable in my own skin. Around this time, I met with the spiritual advisor at my church, and he told me that if I kept a prayer journal that was half as detailed as my food journal, it would change my life. So I took his advice and spent more time turning inward.

Eventually my path led me to become a certified nutritionist. As I studied nutrition, I began to accept the idea that exercising had nothing to do with making myself smaller on the outside—it was to make myself better on the inside. I stopped thinking of exercise as physical and started to see it as *physiological,* or how it affects the body's function, not just the body itself. I shifted my training away from focusing on my appearance and instead focused on my heart and my mind. I started thinking about how my movement could help keep me feeling strong, capable, and balanced. And ultimately, I found gratitude in exercise. Now I'm strong, vibrant, and lean—and I know I'll never weigh less than 140 pounds (and be healthy at the same time). But this body is perfect the way it was made, and I'm keeping it that way!

Christina: People are always asking me what I do to look like me. But the better question for any of us to ask isn't how we can look like someone else, but

"How can I look like the best version of *myself*?" Because even if we followed the same meal plans and the same exercise routine, you and I still most likely wouldn't look exactly the same. That's because **no two bodies are the same**. Cara is the perfect example—she and I follow the same nutrition and exercise program, but we have very different body types. My body will never have the same muscle mass that hers has (unless I get implants in my biceps and glutes). Her body won't have the same measurements as mine unless she has a few ribs removed. Not exactly what either of us wants! So even though you can defy genetics in many ways—eating to stabilize blood sugar and reverse chronic disease is one!—the body you have is ultimately the one you've got. Why waste any time wanting it to be something other than what it is?

Kick It Off with a Sweat Reset

Cara: Just as we shared our meal plan to reboot your body with optimal nutrition, we'll also offer you a companion workout plan. But instead of giving you structured guidelines the way we did with the Reset, these exercises are for you to mix and match in order to find the approach to a movement practice that works best for you. Incorporating these exercises into your routine is a great way to increase the benefits you're already reaping from the Reset. Plus, they help to solve the "am I doing enough?" dilemma. Trust us, they're enough—even just shooting these how-to photos had us working up a sweat! But the best part is that they don't require a gym membership, class fees, or a ton of special equipment—just some free weights, a mat, and a timer—so you can sneak in some exercise any time of day. Let's get after it!

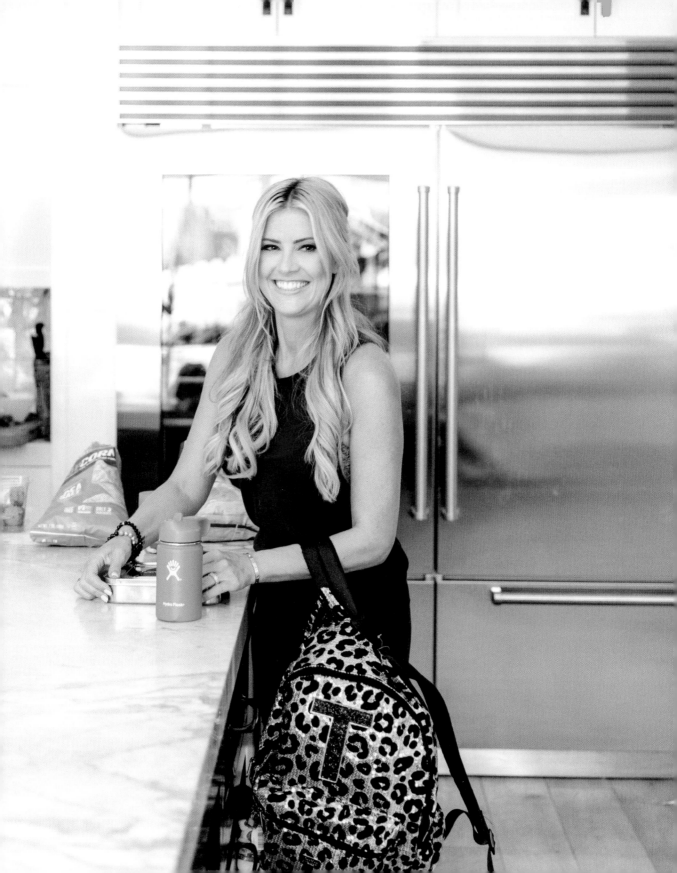

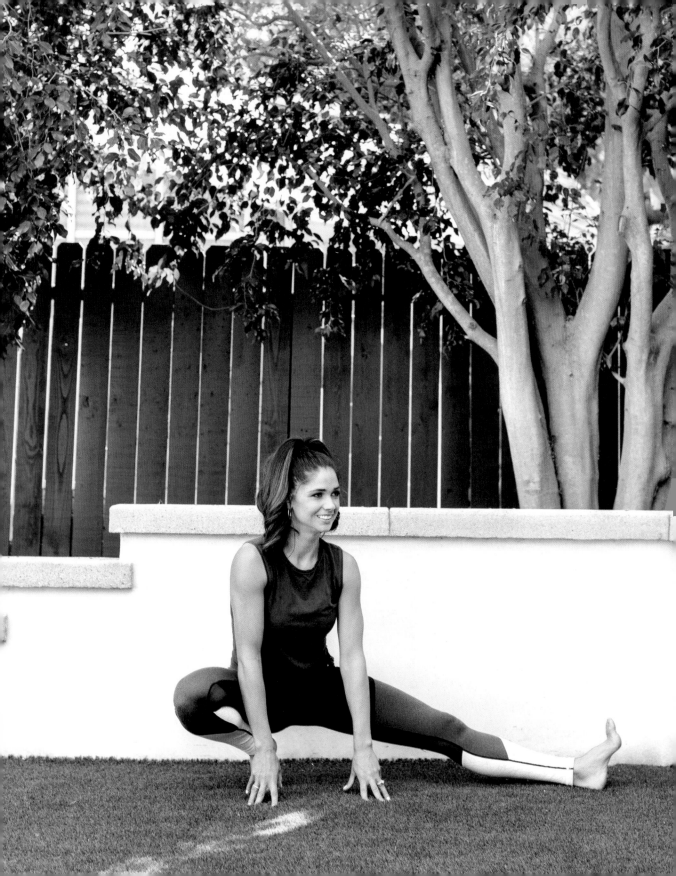

Chapter 5

POWER
TOOLS

Christina: To help you transition to your new workouts, I've teamed up with one of Cara's favorite trainers and friend, Ashley Marks of On Your Marks Fitness, to put together a few basic exercise circuits. Our goal is to first help you find your exercise sweet spot and learn how your body feels when you're not pushing it to the limit or asking too much of it. Then you'll have a foundation for building all other aspects of your fitness, whether you want to make the workouts more or less challenging or combine them with other activities that you love. These workouts are simple, fun, perfect for all fitness levels, and intended to take thirty minutes or less—so you can see that exercise is absolutely something you can fit into your day. These workouts cover upper body, lower body, and cardio + core so that you're getting plenty of variation in a balanced way. That's why this program is awesome for me—I can follow it and know that I'm going to get a great workout and strengthen every part of my body in barely any time. And I don't even need to leave the house! Especially when I feel like I need to hit the reset button, coming back to these moves helps me feel grounded again and gives me amazing workout inspo for getting back on track.

Cara: The plan that follows is totally customizable. You can either do each circut exactly as written, or, if you already have a workout routine in place that follows the general guidelines we've included, feel free to use these exercises to supplement on alternating days. I also encourage you to modify all of these exercises for your fitness level. Every workout has a beginner option listed, and please give yourself permission to follow that if it's appropriate to your body. I can assure you that even the beginner option is going to get you results! Remember, getting your heart rate up to a crazy level isn't the path to success. Conversely, if you feel ready for more of a challenge, then honor that! Here are some ways to customize your workouts:

- CHANGE THE NUMBER OF REPS. A good rule of thumb is that your last 2 to 3 reps should be challenging, but not so hard that you're struggling to keep good form. So if you're barely muscling through the final reps, decrease your reps. Conversely, if you're only feeling slightly challenged, increase your reps.
- CHANGE YOUR RESISTANCE. Same gauge as above—the last 2 to 3 reps should be challenging but not so much so that you're losing correct form. See the next page for tips on how to choose the weight that's right for you.
- CHANGE YOUR INTENSITY. Many workouts include jumping exercises or other high-impact options. If that doesn't work for you, you can modify by opting out of the jumping or substituting other low-impact cardio moves,

such as marching in place or stepping in and out of a gentle squat. Any move that calls for a jump (squat jacks, jumping lunges) can be done by stepping your feet together and then moving on with the exercise. Over time, you can throw in a few reps of the full movement while working up to a full set. Or if it causes you discomfort, stick with the low-impact version—you'll still get your heart rate up and reap the strengthening benefits.

- LISTEN TO YOUR BODY. If something doesn't feel right, it might not be the right exercise for you. Double-check that you're doing the moves with proper form, and if that doesn't resolve the issue, either omit or modify that exercise.

HOW TO CHOOSE THE RIGHT WEIGHTS

This all goes back to the central rule of thumb: The last 2 to 3 reps should be challenging, but not so challenging that your form is compromised. It may take some trial and error at first, and as you get stronger you'll be able to handle heavier weights. Listen to your body! While some workouts call for two sets of weights (lighter and heavier), you could absolutely get away with using just one set of weights and adjusting your reps accordingly.

- Beginners: 3 to 5 pounds is plenty. For exercises that call for a lighter weight, you may even get a challenging enough workout using just your body weight.
- Intermediate: 3 to 5 pounds on the lighter side, 7 or 8 on the heavier.
- Advanced: 5 to 7 pounds on the lighter side, 10 to 12 on the heavier.

UPPER BODY CIRCUIT

EQUIPMENT: 1 or 2 sets of free weights, mat, timer

HOW TO: Warm up with 3 to 5 minutes of cardio of your choice, such as jogging, jumping jacks, or jumping rope.

Once you are warm, set your timer for 2 minutes and complete each exercise in the set, resting for up to 1 minute in between sets. Repeat the circuit 6 times.

BEGINNER'S MODIFICATION: Set your timer for 1 minute and repeat the circuit 3 to 4 times.

| Locomotives | Wide Bicep Curls | Chest Flys |
| Tricep Push-ups | Mountain Climbers | Alternating Overhead Presses |

LOCOMOTIVES

With your feet hip-width apart and knees slightly bent, hinge at the waist, pushing your hips back toward the wall behind you. You want your chest to be parallel to the ground and your back flat. Hold your weights in each hand, with your palms facing each other. Pull your right elbow back, skimming your body with the weight. As you bring it back down to the starting position, you will pull your left elbow back in the same motion. Continue alternating sides, squeezing in your shoulder blades with each movement.

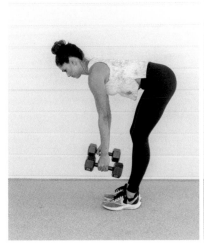
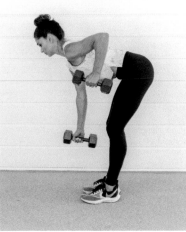
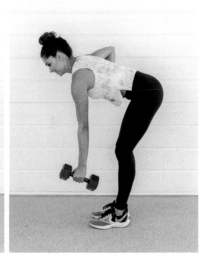

TRICEP PUSH-UPS

Get into high plank position with your hands right underneath your shoulders and your fingers pointed forward, then lower your knees to the ground. Lower your chest to the ground with your elbows pointing behind you. Slowly push your body back up to starting position with arms extended. Be sure to keep your core and hips in line with your shoulders throughout the movement—avoid letting your back dip or hips stick up in the air.

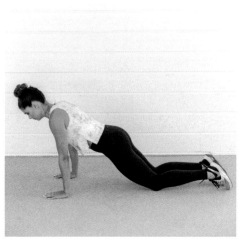 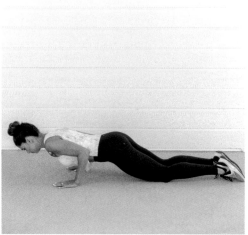

WIDE BICEP CURLS

Stand with your feet hip-width apart and knees slightly bent, your arms at your sides with weights in your hands. Turn your palms to face forward. Keep your elbows in tight to your body and rotate your forearms and hands 45 degrees outward, curling your weights up to your shoulders and back down again while hinging at your elbows. Do not swing your arms.

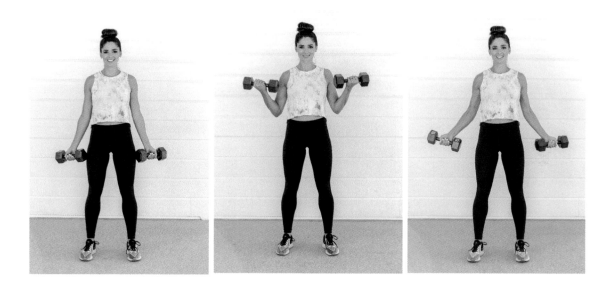

MOUNTAIN CLIMBERS

Start in a high plank position with your hands under your shoulders and your back and hips in line with your shoulders. Bring your right knee in to your chest. Push off your left foot to switch feet in the air.

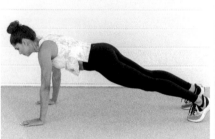 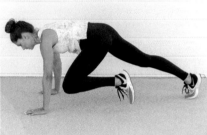 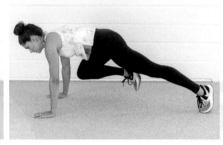

CHEST FLYS

Lie on your back with your knees bent and feet planted on the ground. Begin with your arms extended above your chest, weights in hand, palms facing each other, with a soft bend in your elbows. Bring both arms out to your sides, keeping that soft bend in the elbows. As you exhale, bring your hands back together in starting position. I like to cue this as a big bear hug above your chest.

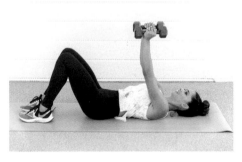 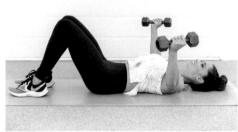

ALTERNATING OVERHEAD PRESSES

Stand with your feet hip-width apart and your knees slightly bent. Hold a weight in each hand and start with your elbows at a 90-degree angle from shoulder height. Your weights should be directly in line with your elbows. Raise your right arm and press the weight overhead. Slowly release back to starting position, and raise your left arm overhead. Focus on coming back to that 90-degree angle after each rep.

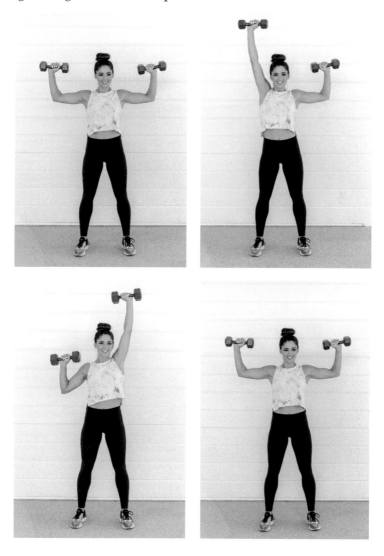

LOWER BODY CIRCUIT

EQUIPMENT: 1 or 2 sets of free weights (I recommend a heavier weight, if you have it), mat

HOW TO: Warm up with 3 to 5 minutes of cardio of your choice, such as jogging, jumping jacks, or jumping rope.

   Once you are warm, repeat each set of exercises for 2 to 3 rounds.

BEGINNER'S MODIFICATION: Complete 1 to 2 rounds of each set and use body weight only.

SET 1

10 Squat Jumps	10 Squat Jumps	25 Plié Squats
25 Goblet Squats	25 Deadlifts	10 Squat Jumps
	10 Squat Jumps	

SET 2

20 Jumping Lunges	20 Jumping Lunges	20 Reverse Lunges
20 Curtsy Lunges	20 Squat Jumps	20 Squat Jumps

SQUAT JUMPS

Stand with your feet shoulder-width apart and squat down, sitting into your heels with your chest open and shoulders back. As you squat, bring your arms behind you. Transfer your weight from your heels to your toes and then jump straight up. Your arms will also swing forward with you as you propel your body upward. If you don't want the high impact of the jump, you may finish on your toes, keeping the same form.

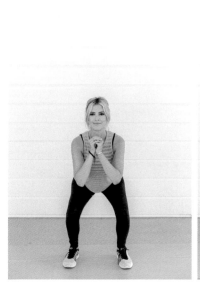 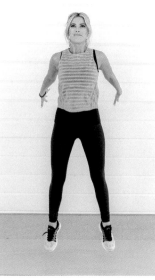 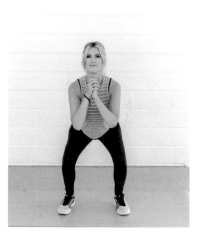

GOBLET SQUATS

Stand with your feet shoulder-width apart and a heavier weight in your hands. Hold your weight at chest level with your palms facing each other and elbows in. Begin squatting by bending your knees and pushing your heels into the floor while keeping your chest open, back flat, and your knees in line with your ankles. At the end of the movement, your quadriceps should be parallel to the ground and elbows inside your knees. Push through your heels to return to standing.

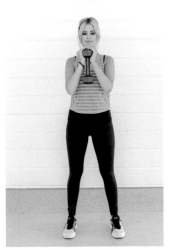
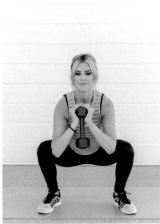
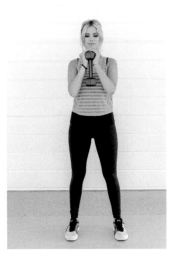

DEADLIFTS

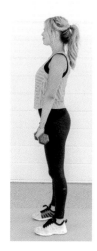
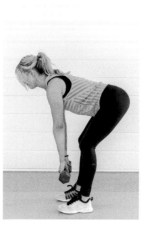
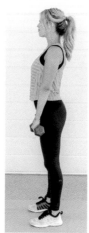

Stand with your feet shoulder-width apart and hold a weight in each hand, arms by your sides. Hinge at your hips with a soft bend in your knees, pushing your glutes back and flattening your low back. Once you are in the hinge position, slowly lower your torso with your weights skimming your shins. You should feel a stretch in your hamstrings as you get lower into the movement. Push through your heels and return to your starting position.

PLIÉ SQUATS

Stand with your feet wider than shoulder-width apart and toes slightly angled out. Lower into a squat, pushing through your heels and ending with your quadriceps parallel to the ground.

ADVANCED VARIATION:

Start from the parallel position and pulse up and down about an inch.

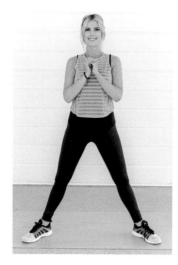
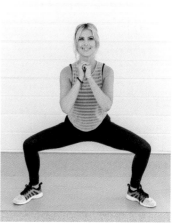

JUMPING LUNGES

Start in lunge position with your right foot forward and right knee bent, keeping your knee above your ankle. Push through your heel and as you jump, switch your lead leg in the air and sink into a lunge with your left foot forward. Continue jumping and switching your lunging leg.

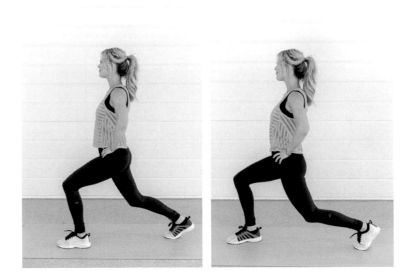

Christina: You'll notice there's no photo of me switching my feet mid-air; that's because I was still recovering from having Hudson and couldn't get the airtime for the shot! Proof that these exercises mean business—and that you should modify them to suit your body's needs.

CURTSY LUNGES

Begin standing with your feet hip-width apart. Step your left foot back and to the side as if you were doing a curtsy, keeping your right foot planted on the ground. Bend your right knee until your quadricep is parallel to the ground. Be sure to sit into your right heel and keep your knee in line with your ankle. Return to the starting position and switch sides.

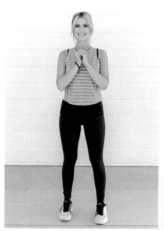 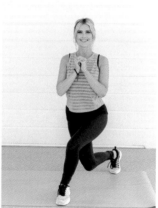 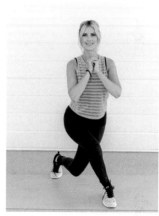

REVERSE LUNGES

Stand with feet shoulder-width apart. Step your right foot straight back and bend your right and left knee while putting your weight into your left heel. Return to starting position by stepping your right foot back to standing and repeat with your left leg.

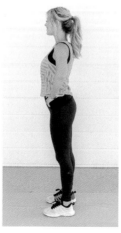 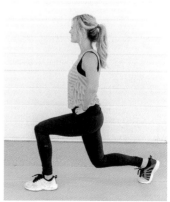

CARDIO AND CORE CIRCUIT

EQUIPMENT: Mat and timer

HOW TO: Warm up with 3 to 5 minutes of cardio of your choice, such as jogging, jumping jacks, or jumping rope.

Once warm, grab your timer and set it for 3 minutes. You will complete each set of specified exercises as many times as you can before your timer goes off, ideally aiming for the noted number of reps. Rest up to 1 minute between each set and repeat once more all the way through.

All rounds in this workout are 3 minutes in total. You may rest up to 1 minute between rounds.

BEGINNERS' MODIFICATION: Complete two 30/30 rounds with a total of 2 minutes per set.

30/30: Squat Jacks + Kickouts
50/10 Leg Raise + Burpees
30/30 Half Burpees + Double Crunches

50/10 Inchworms + Plank Reach
30/30 Froggie Jumps + Bicycle Crunches

50/10/10 Spiderman Planks + Plank Toe Taps + Elbow Up-Downs

ACTIVATING YOUR CORE

Throughout these exercises it's important to keep your core engaged. A common mistake is to think that by sucking in our stomachs we're achieving this. In order to work those deeper abdominal muscles, you need to pull your navel in toward your spine and up toward your rib cage. I tell my clients to pretend someone is trying to punch you in the stomach. If you're lying on the ground, think about pulling your navel to your spine.

If you're postpartum and beginning an exercise regimen, be sure to ask a professional how to reengage your core. Your muscles need to be strengthened more gently than can be accomplished with the exercises in this section. But with some guidance, you'll be ready for mainstream core work in no time!

SQUAT JACKS

Stand with your feet together. Squat before jumping out to a wide jack position and squatting again when you land. Alternate from in and out, always sinking into the squat when your feet hit the ground.

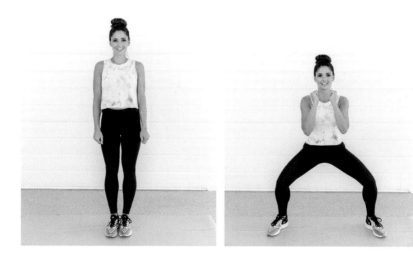

KICKOUTS

Begin from a seated position with your back at a 45-degree angle. Make sure you keep your back flat and your shoulders back. Pick your feet up from the ground and pull your knees into your chest. Push your legs back out to straight and repeat that motion. You may put your hands on the floor behind you for balance.

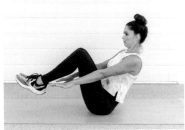 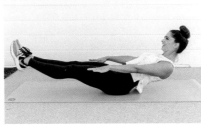 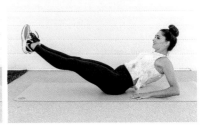

LEG RAISES

Lying on your back, raise both legs up to the sky and, with control, slowly lower them back to a couple inches off the ground, or whatever point you can keep core control. Keep your low back pushed into the ground.

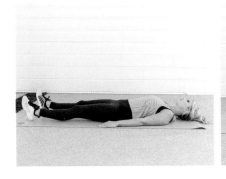 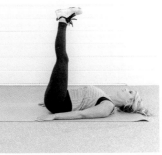 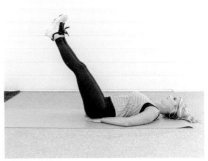

MODIFICATION: *Place your hands under your hips for core support. You may also keep your legs slightly bent if you are a beginner or need more back support.*

BURPEES

Stand with your feet hip-width apart. Put your hands on the ground and either jump or step both feet back behind you so you are in plank position. You can go all the way down touching your chest to the ground, but you may also stop at plank position. Push off the ground and jump or step up.

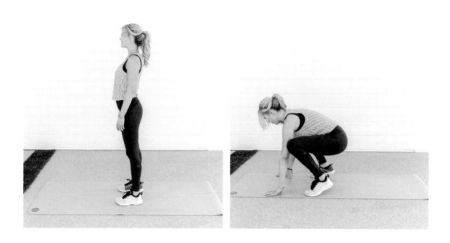

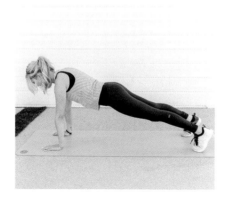

HALF BURPEES

Place your hands on the floor and jump your feet back into a high plank position. Jump your feet back up to elbow-width, planting your feet. Sit back into a deep squat with your chest open. Jump back to plank position.

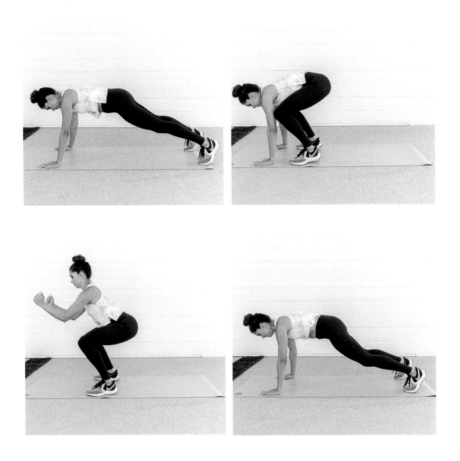

DOUBLE CRUNCHES

Begin by lying on your back with your knees bent and your hands behind your head. Bring your knees to your chest as you lift your shoulders off the ground. Reach your hands toward your knees and then release back to the ground. Keep your back glued to the ground throughout the exercise.

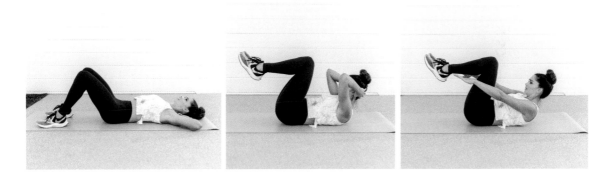

MODIFICATION: *If you have trouble holding the crunch with your feet off the mat or find yourself straining your neck, you can keep your feet on the mat while you reach for your knees.*

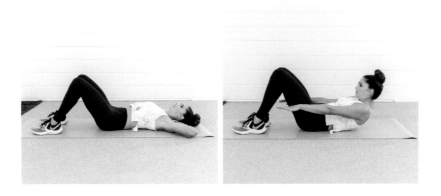

INCHWORMS

Stand at one end of your mat with your feet shoulder-width apart. Bend from your waist and put your hands on the mat. Walk your hands forward until your body is flat in plank position. When your hands are under your shoulders, do the plank reach (see opposite page) on each side then walk your hands back to your toes and return to the upright starting position.

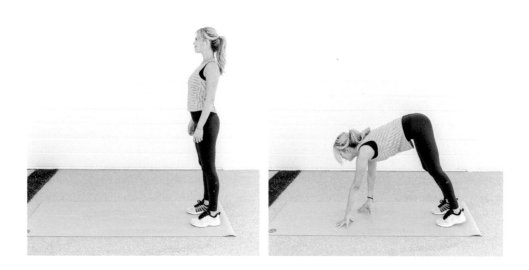

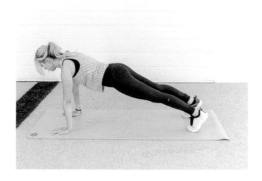

PLANK REACH

Start in a high plank position with your hands under your shoulders and your back and hips in line with your shoulders. Extend one arm straight out and hold for a few seconds before returning to plank. Repeat with the other arm.

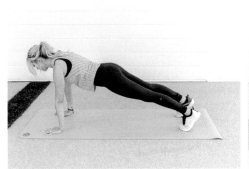 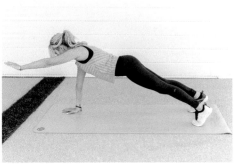

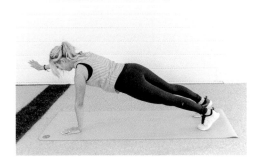

FROGGIE JUMPS

Stand with your feet a little wider than shoulder-width apart, knees bent out like a frog. Perform two 2-footed jumps forward, swinging your arms to help with your momentum. You may either jump or jog backward to return to starting position.

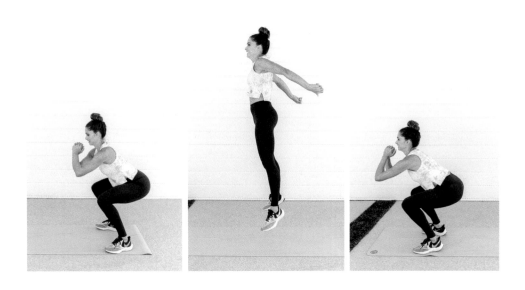

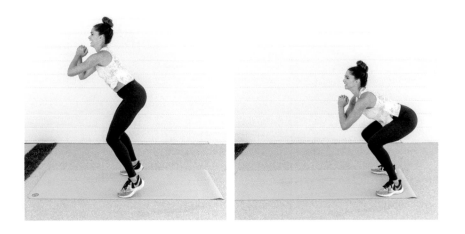

BICYCLE CRUNCHES

Start lying on your back with your hands behind your head and your knees in tabletop position (feet elevated, knees bent). Twist your torso to the left while bringing your left knee in to your chest. Think of your right armpit touching your left knee. Return to starting position and switch sides.

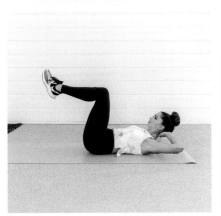 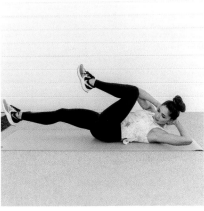

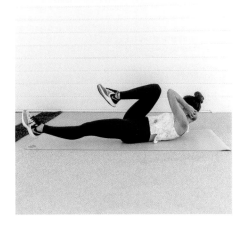

SPIDERMAN PLANKS

Start in high plank position with your hands under your shoulders and your back and hips in line with your shoulders. Starting with your right leg, bring your knee in to the outside of your right elbow, while keeping your hips down. This will isolate your obliques. Bring your right leg back to starting position and alternate sides.

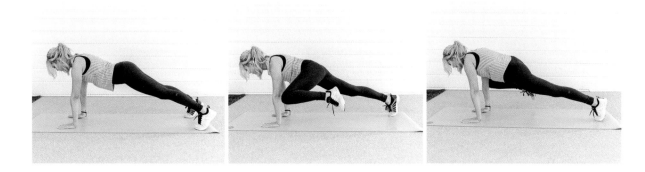

PLANK TOE TAPS

Start in high plank position with your hands under your shoulders and your back and hips in line with your shoulders. Keeping your hips as still as possible, step your feet out to the side one at a time. You will go right leg out, left leg out, right leg in, left leg in.

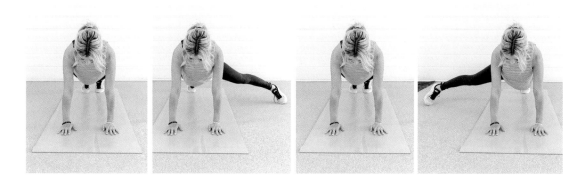

ELBOW UP-DOWNS

Start in a high plank position with your hands under your shoulders and your back and hips in line with your shoulders. Lower your right elbow to the ground followed by your left to put you in a low plank position. Hold for a count or two and then reverse the movement back up to your hands, one arm at a time. Your elbows and hands should stay in line with your shoulders as much as possible.

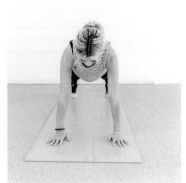 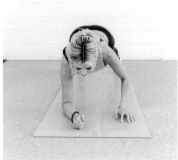 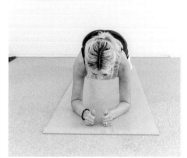

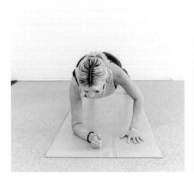 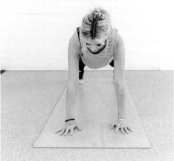

GET YOUR FAMILY IN ON THE FUN

We'll talk more about sneaking in a workout when you're #MommingSoHard in chapter 8, but these workouts are a great way to reap the benefits of exercise while also spending time with your kids. My girls love doing these exercises with me, especially the jumping jacks and burpees. They think it's hilarious and fun, and it changes the experience from something that you have to do into something that you *want* to do. In fact, my kids ask me when it's time for our next living room workout!

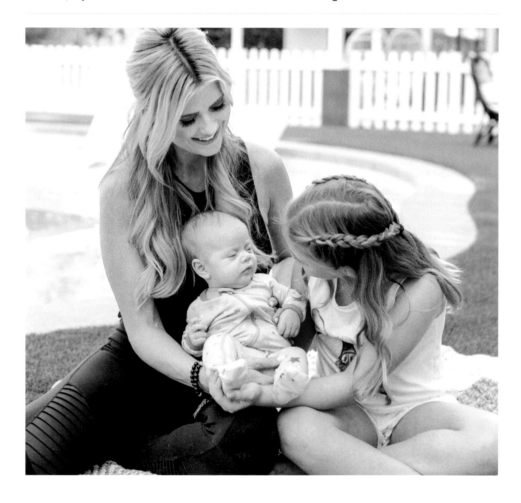

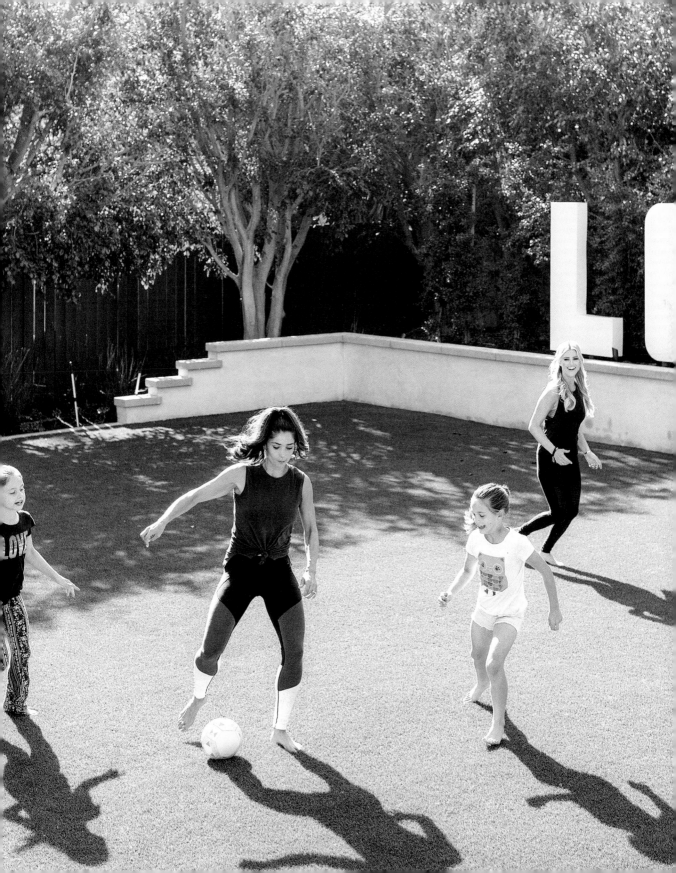

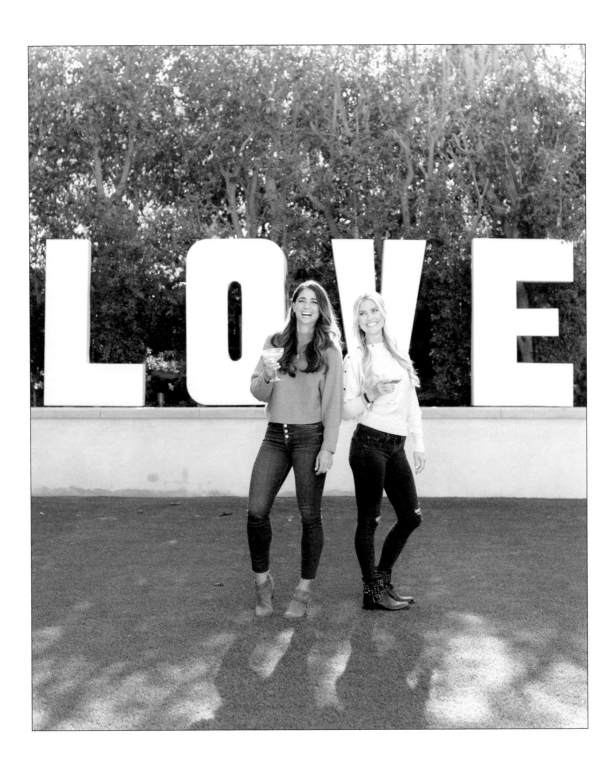

Part III

THE
REWIRE

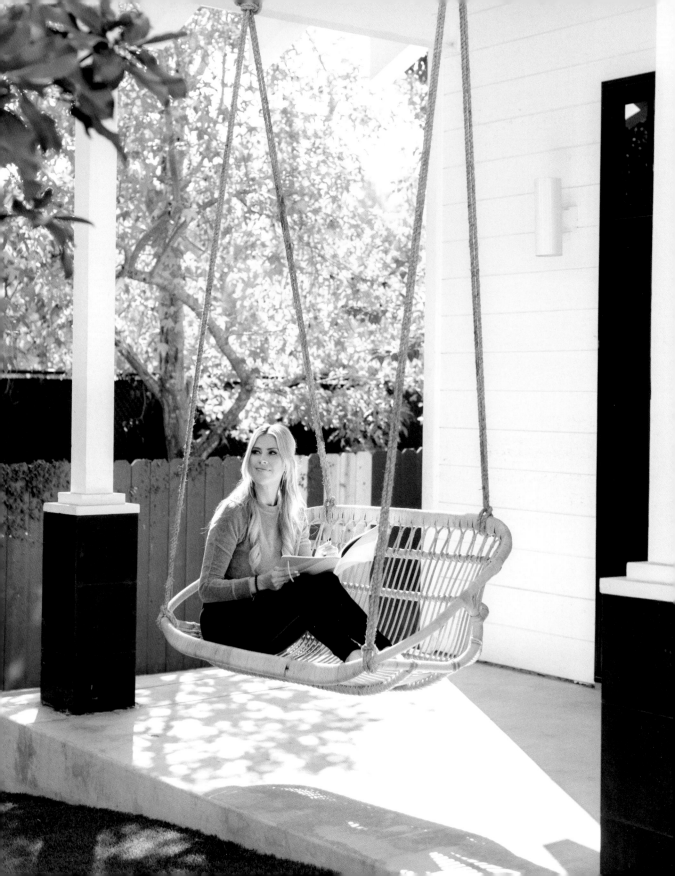

Chapter 6

TURNING
ON THE
LIGHTS

Christina: When we set out to write this book, we were playing around with calling it "Food, Fitness, Family, and Faith." We both knew that we couldn't write about reaching true health and happiness without also talking about faith/spirituality/mindfulness—whatever you want to call it (and we'll help you figure out what to call it in a bit). That's because the thoughts you think, the emotions you experience, and the beliefs you carry around with you have just as big of an impact on your well-being as the food you eat. Thanks to researchers and other experts who specialize in understanding how our bodies and minds work, we now know things like the fact that there's a link between depression and heart disease, that high levels of mental distress are correlated with increased risk of cancer, and that people with depression tend to have more severe diabetes symptoms. On the flip side, practicing mindfulness—or intentionally focusing on the present moment (and accepting it with grace)—can relieve stress, alleviate chronic pain and mood disorders, lower blood pressure, improve sleep, and help to protect against heart disease and alleviate gastrointestinal issues. To sum it up, there is no health without *both* mind and body being onboard.

Cara and I can speak to this firsthand. In our early thirties, stress was a huge issue for us. I had terrible flare-ups of my autoimmune symptoms, to the point where I ended up in the emergency room on multiple occasions. It felt like someone was stabbing me in the stomach, and I would become so nauseous that I couldn't eat. If I did eat, the pain cycle would start all over again. The ER doctors would run tests and scans, and each time they were unable to find anything wrong. Finally, one of them asked me, "Are you experiencing any stress in your life?" (Pause for laughter.) I was going through a divorce, continuing to film my show with my soon-to-be ex, and caring for two young kids. The doctor gave me a prescription for Xanax and some antidepressants. I didn't want to rely on medication if I didn't have to, but at the urging of one of my amazing integrative practitioners, Dr. Peggy Branson, I started to take half a Xanax at bedtime when stress was keeping me up at night so I could finally get some necessary rest. After that, I vowed to start paying as much attention to my mental and emotional health as I was giving to my diet and exercise.

During the next two years I reconnected with my faith, found new power in my positive relationships, disconnected myself from toxic ones, learned how to move and breathe in a restorative way, gave myself permission to take "time-outs," and started dreaming bigger than ever. I was able to put myself back on the path of healing—a path that led me to feeling better than ever before, expanding my professional life (including the book you're holding in your hands!), and meeting the most incredible man and partner and welcoming our baby into the world. And it all started with a little self-love.

Just like a nutritional reset is essential for clearing away the "noise" that can prevent us from fully connecting with our bodies, this chapter is dedicated to another essential piece of the Wellness Remodel philosophy: the mental reset.

Your No-Freak-Out Guide to Stress

Because so many people assume that my life is like some kind of perfect Instagram feed (reason #245 why I have issues with social media, but I'm saving that rant for later!), I want to share just how big of a mess I was before I started getting my stress under control—and before one of my favorite integrative practitioners taught me about my health.

A little while ago I was experiencing an eczema flare-up—something I'd never dealt with before. I asked Cara about it, and she immediately recommended Dr. Kaisa Coppola, an integrative practitioner who was treating Cara's daughter for eczema, and whom Cara trusted with all of her health concerns. When I made the appointment, I really just wanted her to check out my very inflamed, very itchy skin. But Dr. Kaisa suggested a more holistic approach—she also wanted to consider the ways in which other issues I was having might be a factor in my eczema. At the time, I was presenting with symptoms of Hashimoto's disease and polycystic ovary syndrome, plus I was pregnant, so my hormones were going crazy. Her goal was to get to the root of it all, not just look at one individual set of symptoms, so that we could figure out the underlying imbalances and how best to address them.

She ruled out fungal or bacterial issues that may have been affecting my skin, so that tipped her off that there was something my body wasn't handling well internally. And that insight, combined with my autoimmune disease diagnoses, helped us see the big picture: My body was dealing with some pretty serious chronic inflammation.

Dr. Kaisa explained to me that inflammation gets a bad rap, but it's actually an essential function of the body's immune system. It's how your body responds to injury or infection, signals for necessary repairs on damaged tissue, and defends itself against viruses and bacteria. Inflammation becomes a problem when it is chronic—when the body feels it is constantly under attack and responds accordingly. That's when you start seeing symptoms such as body pain, fatigue, sudden weight gain/loss, mood disorders, skin disorders, and, eventually, autoimmune disorders.

So Dr. Kaisa wanted to take a closer look at what factors in my life were causing my symptoms to flare up and, most urgently, this rash. To start, we looked at food—which is where she begins with all of her clients. Using an elimination diet (like our Reset in chapter 3) and blood work, she was able to see that even the tiniest bit of gluten was causing a lot of inflammation. I very quickly took that out of my diet, but there was something else that we needed to explore, which Dr. Kaisa explained was a health issue for the majority of her patients: stress.

Stress: the CliffsNotes Version

I'm not a doctor, but thanks to Dr. Kaisa and all of her insight on the topic of stress, I can sometimes sound (a little bit) like one. This is how Dr. Kaisa broke it down for me: Stress, like inflammation, can actually be a good thing in the short term. As humans, we evolved in a dangerous world, and we needed to respond quickly to the environment around us. If you encountered a predator, then your sympathetic nervous system—part of your central nervous system—would tell your adrenal glands to pump out stress hormones like epinephrine, adrenaline, and cortisol. You would then enter "fight or flight" mode, meaning you could make a split-second decision about whether it was beneficial to freeze or run. This would cause your heart to pump more quickly, your breathing to speed up, your muscles to tense, your digestive function to pause, and your blood pressure to rise. Eventually, when your body recognized that the threat had passed, the *parasympathetic* nervous system—the sympathetic nervous system's cool, calm counterpart—would kick in, and you'd enter "rest and digest" mode—your body's happy place where everything is in balance, i.e., homeostasis.

The issue is that even though our prehistoric predators are extinct, our prehistoric stress response remains very much alive. So while the majority of our day-to-day "threats" aren't actually life-threatening (traffic, e-mail, social media posts), our stress response still kicks in. So many people are walking around with their sympathetic nervous system constantly on high alert. When that happens, your body is going to do its best to reenter homeostasis—and it most frequently does that by changing up your hormones. If cortisol is high, then often your body tries to balance this out by keeping other hormones, such as progesterone, low. Over time, the hormones that are instructed to lie low lose their function. Dr. Kaisa says she sees patients who have issues with their thyroid, blood sugar, and polycystic ovary syndrome—but thyroid, insulin, and estrogen production isn't the core issue—cortisol is.

One of the most important things you can do for your health is to manage your stress, and that starts with recognizing the symptoms. These days everyone struggles with busy-itis. We all brag or complain about how busy we are, or we think that it's normal to multitask and never stop working or moving. Then we wonder why we're walking around inflamed, bloated, cranky, and tired! So start by checking in: how do you feel?

Do you experience any of these symptoms?

- Fatigue
- Brain fog
- Bloat or other digestion issues
- Headaches
- Aches and pains
- Skin issues (rashes, breakouts)
- Irregular periods
- Irritability or mood disorders such as depression or anxiety
- Low libido

We've all seen these signs, some of us more than others. They're your body's way of telling you that something isn't quite right. If these symptoms haven't gone away after addressing your relationship with food, then it's time to start thinking about your relationship with stress.

I believe we are all meant to be creators *and* we were meant to be servers—whether it's your community, your family, the universe, God, mankind, the planet, whatever. When our bodies are balanced and our thoughts are centered and peaceful, then we get to serve. We have energy to give. If everything is in harmony, then we get to be expansive, we get to be creative. And we get to create.

BOX BREATHING

This is an amazing tool that Dr. Kaisa taught me because one of the most powerful ways to bring your body back into a parasympathetic state is with breath. You can do this anywhere, any time of day, and it takes about ninety seconds. It's an opportunity for you to leave behind what's happened and set an intention for what comes next. I particularly love to do this practice when I'm transitioning between parts of my day, like when I'm waiting in my car to pick up my kids from school. I take a moment to breathe, leave my work at the office, and then resolve to be a focused, present, patient parent.

How to practice Box Breathing: Take a deep inhale for a count of your choice. If you're just beginning, you may want to start with 5. If you're experiencing shortness of breath because of stress, start smaller, like with 3. Hold your breath for the same count. Release the breath for the same count, and again hold for the same count (like a box with four equal sides). Repeat. Try working up to a count of 10 seconds, for 10 breaths.

Keeping the Faith

Once Cara and I realized how big of an impact stress had on our health, we both vowed to do our best to slow down (as much as possible), breathe more, and see the beautiful things in our crazy lives. We'll be talking more about the small practices we use on a day-to-day basis to hit the refresh button, but there's one really big thing that we both do almost every moment of every day: We have faith.

Before I jump into this section, I want to be totally clear: Faith isn't necessarily *religious*. For Cara and me, our faith is in God. For friends of mine, it's universe or spirit. What we all have in common is that we believe that there's a higher power that's bigger than we are. I don't want to get all woo-woo on you, but that belief is a huge part of what keeps me feeling grounded and centered. Faith—combined with therapy and spiritual healing—is what has helped me pick myself off the floor, breathe in new lightness and positivity, and reach my biggest, dreamiest goals. And by extension, it has transformed my health.

I didn't grow up religious at all. I pretty much just went to church when people were baptized or if there was a big holiday. But during my divorce, when I felt so helpless and alone and like I couldn't deal with it by myself anymore, I tried talking to God. I started going to church, and I started praying. I began seeing messages everywhere that let me know that I was on the right path, and that I wasn't alone. Over time, my prayers started to be answered, in little and big ways. It was such a relief to know that not all the decisions were mine, that the burdens weren't mine either, and that there was light at the end of the tunnel. I felt so much better, so much more connected. It even gave me the confidence to take risks in my career.

But the most powerful outcome of all was how this newfound faith affected my stress levels. When I opened my eyes to the miracles in everyday life, I naturally felt gratitude. I found that I was less focused on the bad things and wasn't as caught up in anxiety over what I couldn't control. No matter your faith or beliefs, I challenge you to try to recognize the positive things in your life, and to pay as much (ideally more) attention to them as you do the negative things. You will naturally experience more gratitude, and when that happens, the stressful stuff doesn't seem as stressful anymore. We'll talk more about some great practices you can use to cultivate gratitude in the next chapter, but for now, consider simple new habits like journaling about what you're grateful for before you go to bed, or taking a minute—before you check your phone!—to list five things you're grateful for when you first wake up in the morning.

This is not to say that life won't hand you challenges, or that a higher power can take away all of your struggles. That's part of the process! Experiences that knock us down, challenge our faith, or cause us pain will inevitably happen. But if you can meet those challenges with an open heart and the belief that maybe—just maybe—something positive may come from them (no matter how hard you may have to look), then the world becomes a gentler place to live in. When you do your best to keep moving forward and treat others with respect and kindness, I believe that eventually you'll start to notice amazing synchronicities that confirm that you're most definitely not on your own, that you got this, and that good things are coming for you. And when you have that kind of reassurance, you'll be coming from a stronger, more empowered place to go out into the world and make your own magic.

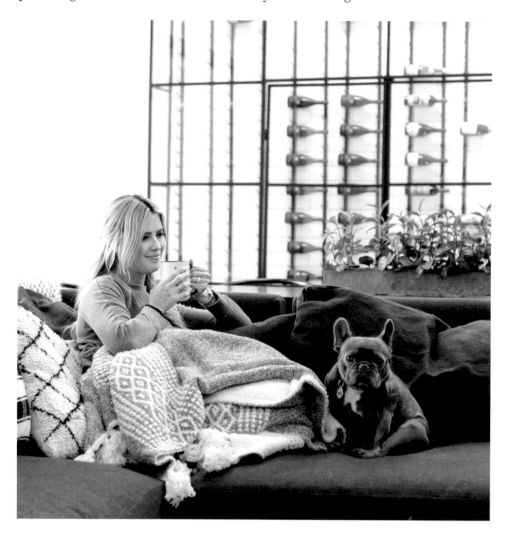

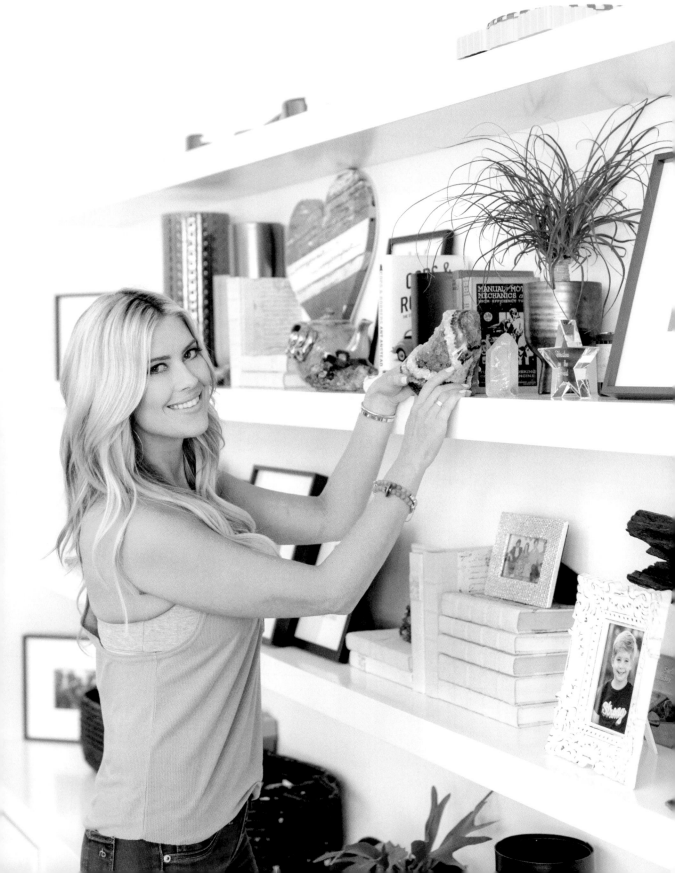

Chapter 7

FINDING YOUR GLOW

Cara: Ironically, stress was one of the things that helped Christina and me become so close. Around the same time that she was navigating her divorce and low moments in her health, I was also struggling. I was dealing with all the demands of my growing business while also being the on-call parent for four kids—and my relationship with my husband was bearing the brunt of it. It seemed like I could never get on top of everything—like I was constantly cleaning up spilled water while my cup continued to overflow. I started to see physical manifestations of stress show up, too. I would get intense stomach-aches and break out in hives, my head would feel like it was spinning, and I could never catch my breath. I felt like I was breathing through a coffee straw for an entire year.

As women and as moms, we're so good at convincing ourselves that our needs aren't important, that our kids, our partners, our coworkers, our bosses, and our friends need us more than we need ourselves. I was caught in that cycle, and my body was basically screaming for help. Christina was the one who called me out on it. She told me I needed to slow down, take some breaths, and then get some support. At the time my daughter was seeing Dr. Kaisa for some health issues, and I decided it was time to make myself an appointment.

Dr. Kaisa basically changed my life (which is why I later recommended Christina see her, too!). She helped me understand that stress was the culprit behind my physical symptoms, and that I couldn't start to feel better until my body got the clear message from my mind that I was happy and safe. She gave me tools to break the stress cycle, which then helped me see that my symptoms were a physiological response to stress, and that actually, at my core, I was happy and safe. It was the demands of such a busy life that hijacked my nervous system and caused me to feel out of control. But the best part of doing this work with Dr. Kaisa was that, like Christina, I started to feel more gratitude. And when I started to open up and lead with gratitude—recognizing simple joys that I was taking for granted, being thankful for lessons that challenges taught me—the world opened up to me, too. I felt more connected to my husband, more present for my kids, and more available to my clients. I finally felt a deep-rooted sense of peace and joy.

If you can relate to my experience, or if you're experiencing symptoms like unexplained weight gain, aches and pains, a mind that won't settle, digestive problems, and issues with sleep, then chances are you've hit a level of stress that your body wasn't built to handle. No guilt or blame! There's a lot to be stressed about and stress is a part of life—it's never going to go away entirely. Whether it's the big stuff like divorce or financial struggles, or little stuff like getting through your to-do list or getting the kids to school on time—it is a constant. So instead of avoiding stressful situations, we have to learn healthy habits for living with stress.

Luckily, there are a lot of simple tools you can use to help improve your mental and emotional health and make you more resilient in the face of stress. Whether it's reading a book, spending some time outside, turning to prayer and/or meditation, listening to a podcast that inspires you, or calling a babysitter for an hour so you can just *be* (or locking yourself in a closet for ten minutes—whatever works!), it all adds up. It not only helps you take a breather and check in to the present moment, but doing things that calm your mind also sends powerful ripples through your body that help bring healing and calm to every cell. That's why we wanted to dedicate a chapter to the soul-soothing, mind-expanding, spirit-brightening techniques you can use to manage stress.

Clear Your Mind

Christina: When I was at my lowest, most stressed-out point, all I found myself wishing for again and again was *peace.* I was holding on to so much anxiety, and I was filling my mind with other peoples' expectations. I wanted to feel calm, even if it was just for ten minutes. That's when I discovered the transformative power of meditation.

I had pretty low expectations at first because I'd never meditated before and it sounded boring (and hard). Also, who has the time to sit still and *not* think?! But I did some research and was intrigued by the benefits. I read that meditation helps the parasympathetic nervous system (helping it to be less reactive to stressful situations) click on, and also that meditation can literally transform your brain, helping it to be less reactive to stressful situations. In fact, meditating regularly can actually change the structure of your brain, bulking up the parts that are responsible for learning and decreasing the area that perceives anxiety and stress.

I decided to give it a try and downloaded a few apps, including Headspace, Meditate, and Buddhify, and chose a practice that was no more than ten to twenty minutes. Every time I used the Headspace app, the narrator would ask me to do a body scan, moving slowly up my body from my feet to my head. At first, all I could feel was the stress and anxiety, and my brain would be going a million miles an hour with negative thoughts. But after a few months of regular practice, I realized that my mind had quieted. My body felt relaxed, and I felt more present and at peace. Now I rely on regular meditation to keep me feeling good mentally *and* physically every day.

Yin Yoga

As I was looking for ways to reduce my stress levels, a friend of mine recommended that I try something called yin yoga. In my mind, I was envisioning a rigorous workout, and I was ready to get my sweat on. But the woman who showed up at my door—Natalie Rodriguez, who has become a good friend—wasn't wearing athletic attire; she was carrying a sound bowl. At the time, though, I had no idea what she had in her hands or what she was doing, and when she asked me to lie down and think about my life while she sang and made noises with the bowl, I thought she was crazy. But I wanted to be polite, so I lay down and she began to do her thing.

And then I started to cry.

Now, I'm not a crier; I'm not someone who usually exhibits a lot of outward emotion. But as I lay in restorative poses while she repeated mantras or used aromatherapy with essential oils along with the sound bowl (the sound vibrations it produces, I learned, dial both your brain and nervous system into a more relaxed, meditative frequency), I experienced such a huge *release*. It was like a soul cleanse. Our first two sessions basically consisted of me lying on the floor with tears streaming down my face—it felt amazing and was unlike anything I'd ever done before.

So, what is yin yoga? Many people have heard of restorative yoga, which is a 100-percent passive version of the type of yoga you do at most studios. In restorative yoga, you use props like pillows to relax into a handful of poses that allow you to rest your body and mind completely. Yin yoga is similar to restorative yoga, but the

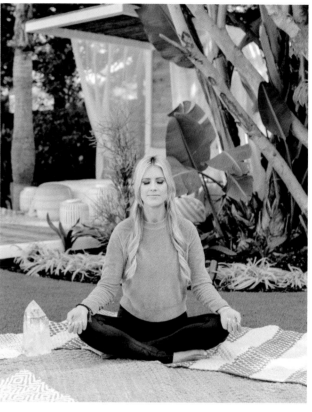

idea of yin is to be nurturing to the body while still actively stretching. It's about reaching your limits with the intent of stretching ligaments, tendons, and fascia. You can achieve this by approaching the discomfort of a pose or stretch and then using props to hold that stretch with as little effort as possible. The idea is to work through the discomfort and find peace in doing so.

Now I practice yin yoga once a week, every week, and it's as powerful as any medicine I could take. I'm able to sleep more soundly, focus my mind and attention so that outside circumstances don't affect my sense of peace, and set healthy boundaries. I highly recommend seeking out a studio or practitioner who offers a yin class, or even finding one online. Once you know the basics, it's easy to do at home on your own.

ESSENTIAL OILS FOR ENHANCING A YIN YOGA PRACTICE

During our sessions, Natalie and I worked on my heart chakra, which is associated with balance, calmness, and serenity. We used essential oils to deepen our connection with this energy point. Here's a quick run-down on the oils I like to use:

LEMON: I love how sweet, refreshing, and clean this scent is, which also happens to benefit the vascular system—think circulation, blood pressure, and lymphatic detoxification. According to Natalie, it also lightens confusion, brings clarity, and uplifts the spirit. Lemon is particularly helpful in opening the heart chakra to self-love and self-nurturing.

EUCALYPTUS: Eucalyptus symbolizes openness and freedom. It is stimulating, decongestive, and soothing to the lungs. It opens the chest and allows the flow of energy through the heart chakra. Eucalyptus has been used to treat respiratory ailments such as bronchitis and colds. On the psychological level, eucalyptus is a central nervous system sedative and calms and uplifts the spirit.

LAVENDER: Lavender is an adaptogenic essential oil, which means it works wherever it is needed. It is universal for all seven chakras and works to calm strong emotions, release pent-up energy, and encourage the life force to flow through the body. As a heart chakra essential oil, lavender helps us to relax, let go of the stress response, and release fear. In this relaxed state we can connect with the heart center and open up to more love.

Using Mantras to Deepen Your Practice

When I first started working with Natalie, the mantra we used was "peace begins with me," which focuses on the idea that in order to achieve peace amid the chaos, you have to begin within. We may not be able to control our outside circumstances, but we have a choice within ourselves in how we choose to respond or react to any given situation. To bring intention to this mantra, we incorporated finger positioning that changes with each word.

Incorporating a mantra into your practice is a great way to further slow down your mind and be fully present on the yoga mat, especially when you incorporate the hand movements. Here's how to do it: In a seated position with your palms up on your knees, say the mantra in your mind. Now bring your hands into it: Peace (thumbs to index fingers) Begins (thumbs to middle fingers) With (thumbs to ring fingers) Me (thumbs to pinkies). Another mantra you might use for a practice focusing on the heart chakra could be: *"I give and receive unconditional love."*

Sometimes I also like to practice a loving-kindness mantra that sends compassion to a loved one, to myself, and out into the world. Here's how I do it: Place a few drops of essential oil in the palms of your hands and rub them together in front of your nose to create an aromatic experience. Cup your hands in front of your face and breathe in with intention. Repeat the following mantra using "I," then "you," and then "we": *"May _____ be filled with loving kindness, May _____ be well, May _____ be peaceful and at ease, may _____ be happy."*

Creating a High-Vibration Space with Crystals

Crystals are some of my favorite healing tools for mind, body, and spirit. In addition to being beautiful in their unique shapes and colors, they help me channel the kind of energy that I want to surround myself with—and deflect the energy that I don't. Even though each type of crystal has its own special properties and powers, I like to think of all my crystals as protective shields that wrap me in love and security. I get that for some people all this talk of "energy" and "vibes" might feel a little abstract or even silly. And that's okay—not everything is for everyone. I can only speak my own healing journey. For me, crystals remind me to be present with what I want more of in my life and what no longer serves me. And that kind of mindfulness is exactly what helps manifest love, happiness, health, and all the other good things we all want and deserve.

Since there are so many different kinds of crystals, I encourage you to seek out the ones that speak most to you. In the meantime, here are my top five:

BLACK TOURMALINE

This is a powerful stone for protection against negative energy of all kinds, including "psychic attacks." This is when someone else—whether intentionally or not—is sending negative energy your way. It usually manifests as bad dreams, a bout of bad luck, or feeling physically drained when you're around this person. Tourmaline not only helps to deflect the attacks but also to ground you again so that you're no longer influenced by that negativity. I keep four of these stones in the corners of my bedroom and carry one in my purse at all times. If you've watched *Flip or Flop*, then you've seen me wearing black tourmaline bracelets in every episode. My husband also carries one in his cargo pants at work!

ROSE QUARTZ

This is the love crystal. It opens the heart to promote unconditional love and positive energy to promote deep inner healing. I have a rose quartz on my nightstand and love giving this crystal as a gift to my friends looking for love.

CLEAR QUARTZ

My favorite stone to decorate the house with! I love the way it looks—it really complements my décor—and it's also a stone that lets in love and light. It looks positively angelic when the light reflects off of it. Clear quartz is queen of manifestation—it helps your raise your vibration (as in, it makes sure your messages are received by your higher power loud and clear) and is also the ultimate healing stone. If you go with only one stone, consider making it a clear quartz.

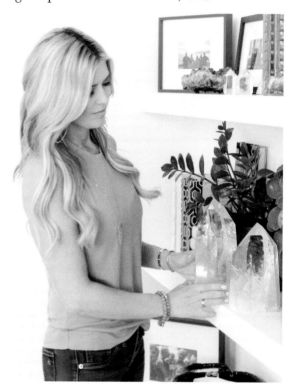

AMETHYST

Amethyst activates your intuition while simultaneously calming your mind. It empowers you to trust your gut. When my new show, *Christina on the Coast*, got picked up—a great example of the good that comes when you wait patiently for the right opportunity—I gifted myself my angel wings amethyst. They sit to the left of my bed, where I can see them when I first wake up in the morning.

HEMATITE

Hematite is the ultimate grounding stone, helping you maintain balance, get rid of negative energy, and amplify your energy so that it vibrates at the highest level of love and light. It also happens to be my favorite color, a beautiful shade of slate/silver.

Get Some Rest

During times of stress, sleep is the first thing that goes. I'll wake up at 2 AM, head spinning, thinking about all kinds of useless crap, and then not be able to fall back asleep. It becomes a vicious cycle because the less sleep you get, the harder it is to cope with stress, and so on. That's why Cara recommended that I create a bedtime relaxation routine to fall asleep and *stay* asleep.

At first when Cara proposed a structured end-of-day ritual, I was like *No. Way. I don't have time for that!* But then I thought about how important a bedtime routine is to my kids—it helps them relax and wind down and I thought, why not give myself a chance to experience the same benefits? So I created my own version: taking a bath, followed by some time reading a good book, talking with my husband, and meditating with Headspace. I also began taking a few tablets of magnesium about thirty minutes before bed, which Dr. Kaisa recommended to me. I think they help to quiet my racing thoughts and make me fall asleep faster. While I'm not always able to do my whole pre-sleep regimen every night, I do keep the basic elements consistent, and I go back to my full routine anytime I feel stress creeping in or have trouble sleeping.

Cara: Sleep isn't just crucial for being resilient to stress, it's crucial for just about every element of your health. When you get the sleep you need, your brain can flush itself of damaging toxins (which have been linked to dementia), your metabolism reregulates, and you'll feel more productive and positive. You may even see a reduction in symptoms from chronic heath issues, thanks to the fact that more and better sleep contributes to a stronger immune system as well as a better-managed stress response, which leads to less body-wide inflammation. The converse is also true. When you don't get the sleep you need, not only will you feel run-down and foggy, but a consistent lack of sufficient sleep puts you at an increased risk for weight gain, depression and anxiety, high blood pressure, and even Alzheimer's disease.

How Much Sleep Do I Need?

Ideally you would get seven to nine hours of sleep every night, although I have some clients who do well with just six hours. It comes back to recognizing what works for you and your body, as Christina has discovered with her sleep routine. That said, I'm more interested in having you commit to *consistency* than to commit to a number. If you can commit to getting to bed by 10 PM every night, then commit to that—and see if you can sleep until 6 AM for eight great hours of rest. If you can only get seven hours, don't beat yourself up. Try to feel grateful for the restorative sleep you got and see what adjustments you can make to get more sleep the next night.

Tools for Peaceful Sleep:

- UNPLUG: When 7 PM rolls around, my in-box is closed and my phone is on airplane mode. Screen time—specifically social media—can send you reeling in an unhealthy direction, which is the last thing you need before bed. Also, the blue light emitted from screens (including phones, computer monitors, tablets, and televisions) can impair your body's production of melatonin. No, that's not just a supplement you can buy at the drugstore to help you sleep, it's an actual hormone that your body produces in order to regulate your sleep/wake cycle. See, your body knows when it's time to sleep—when it's dark out. As your eyes begin to perceive less light, the brain is prompted to produce more melatonin. This sends the signal to your body that it's time to slow down. But if you're exposed to screens right before bed, your body doesn't get the message that it's time to start shutting down for the day. This leads to less melatonin production, poor-quality sleep, and ultimately, it can throw off your entire sleep/wake cycle and set you up for the chronic health conditions that come with it.

- WELCOME GRATITUDE: Something that helps me fall asleep is lying in bed and thinking of five to ten things I'm grateful for. It calms my mind and tells my body that I'm ready for sleep. These things can be as tiny as having all the ingredients in the fridge for my favorite breakfast the next morning, or bigger and more substantial, like my children's health. And they don't all have to be good things. Doors get shut all the time, and I say, *Thank you for shutting the door; that clearly wasn't meant for me.* Here's a simple gratitude mantra that I use before I drift off: "Please open all the doors that will bring peace and prosperity into my life, and please shut all doors that will cause anxiety and tension."

- JOURNAL: When it's time to sleep, my head is always spinning with all the things I didn't get gone done during the day. And sometimes that nagging feeling can wake me up in the middle of the night and make it really hard to fall back asleep. Then I started journaling, and it was like all those crazy, manic thoughts just drained out of my brain and onto the paper. Whether I'm making to-do lists or just reflecting on my day, the simple process of writing it down means there's less work for my brain to do when it's time to shut off and relax.

Know When to Connect . . .

Cara: When my youngest daughter was only a few months old, I had plans to go on a couple's trip to Mexico. I had gigantic boobs, a swollen tummy, and I was dealing with some major postpartum body blues. I told Christina that I was thinking about bailing on the trip, and she reminded me that I really needed this time to get away and be with my husband. And then, even though she also had her hands full with her own infant at the time, she went through her closet and packed at least ten outfits—cover-ups, bathing suits, daytime and nighttime clothes, hats, and bags and dropped off a neatly packed suitcase at my house. I'm pretty sure there were even books in there for me to read. I mean, who does that?! It turns out, a really great friend does.

Christina: A good friend is like free therapy. It's someone who will build you up in a world where everyone's tearing one another down, and it's someone you can vent to and lean on. Cara has been that person for me for the past six years, giving me love, reassurance, and strength when I've needed it most. And in return, I get to be there for her. When we're together, we both feel more alive. We don't even have to say anything to know exactly what's going on with each other—we can feel the lightness or the heaviness. That kind of connection is not only medicine for the soul, it's healing for the body, too. When you share the things that make you feel worried, angry, or overwhelmed, then you release those emotions from your body and prevent them from turning into physical stress that can make you sick.

. . . And When to Disconnect

Christina: As important as it is to have positive people in your life who bring you happiness, it's just as important to let go of the people who cause you distress. Sometimes we give too much energy to people who are toxic for our well-being. How do you know who those people are? You'll feel tired, drained, or just a little off after spending time with them. Unfortunately, you can't always cut the energy suckers out of your life completely. And also unfortunately, you can't always solve the situation by talking things out with them or setting boundaries (though that's always a great place to start!). But you can protect yourself from their negative vibes—something I've gotten very good at doing over the years, out of necessity for my health and my sanity. When I stopped letting other people's negative energy sludge up my own light, I felt so much better—and people started saying I looked different, too! Brighter, younger, more vibrant. Here's what you can do to clear someone's negative energy:

- BURN SOME SAGE: Also called "smudging," the practice of burning a bundle of dried sage leaves (aka, a smudge stick) is an ancient spiritual ritual that many Native American tribes have practiced. It's believed to purify or cleanse a space of negative energy and has also been shown to alleviate stress, improve sleep, and generally lift the spirits.

  Start by opening all the windows and doors on one side of the house (so the negative energy goes out and can't come back in). Light your sage, let it burn for about 20 seconds, and then gently blow out the flame so that you see only orange embers on one end. There's more than one way to clear your space, but I like to start at the front door. I say a prayer for peace, love, and protection of the house and call in archangel Michael to ask for his assistance in getting rid of any unwanted energy in the space.

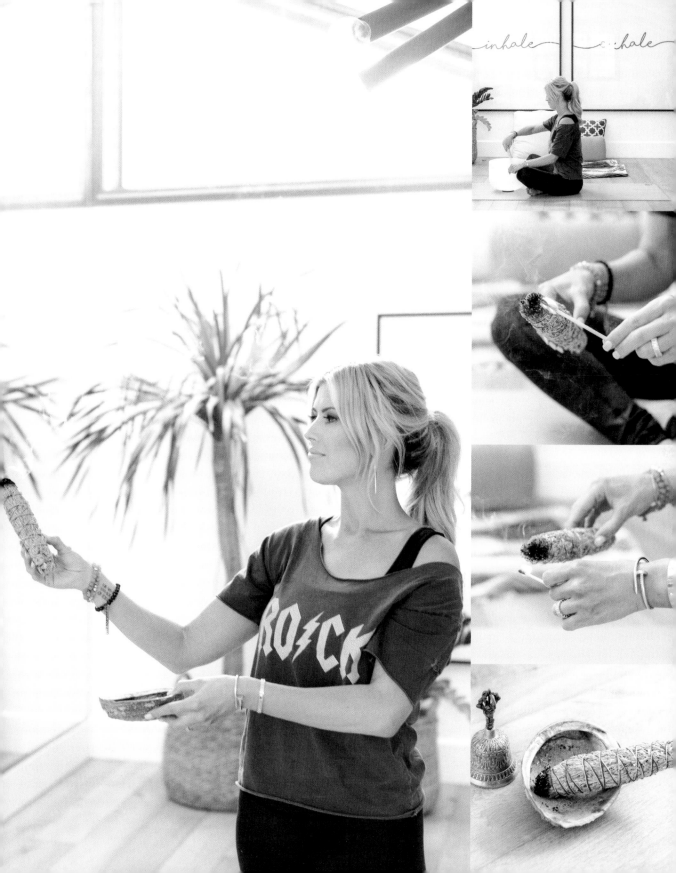

inhale   hale

Then, working one room at a time, I walk around each space, moving the sage counterclockwise and saying out loud that no negative energy is allowed here, only peace, love, and joy. When you've done every room, tap out the sage to extinguish it in an abalone shell or heatproof bowl until no more smoke is coming off of it. After that, you're welcome to do what I do to seal in the practice, which is to go clockwise in each room, ringing a bell in the corners three times and asking for peace, love, and protection.

- PRACTICE A MANTRA: Another way to deal with negative energy is to create a mantra you can say—out loud or just in your head—any time you feel that person affecting you. Here's an example: *I'm sorry for your suffering; it wasn't my fault* or *I'm a sovereign being of light: my energy belongs to me and you have no authority here.*

- OFFER GRATITUDE for one positive thing that person brings to you and your life. I know it sounds counterintuitive, and it might be impossible in some cases, but oftentimes it's easier than you think to find a tiny fleck of something good that's come from your relationship. It can even be recasting a negative like *I'm grateful this person has shown me what I don't want in a relationship. They've helped me get clear on what my needs are and how to protect them.* A little bit of gratitude can go a very long way in releasing someone's negative hold on you.

Social Media Detox

Let's be honest—pretty much all of us are tied to our feeds and our devices. I get that social media offers a way for us to express ourselves and feel more connected . . . but let's be honest once again—is it really doing that for you?

It's so easy to get sucked into these fantasies that people very intentionally create, only posting the best pictures of themselves and making it look like life is nothing but rosé and smoothie bowls. We just end up comparing ourselves and feeling like we're always coming up short. And that's not just my personal opinion—it's backed up by science! Studies have proven that there's a link between social media use and feelings of depression, anxiety, and loneliness in addition to lower self-esteem and even suicidal thoughts.

About a month ago, I decided I wanted to get off that hamster wheel, so I went on a two-week social media detox. I deleted the apps off my phone, and while I was at it, I set a goal to check my e-mail only every two hours, with five minutes to respond. I even set a timer to hold me to it. In addition to clearing up space in my brain and giving me back energy that I'd been spending on creating posts, it also made me realize how much time I was spending aimlessly scrolling through my phone when I could be doing so many other, more productive things. In those two weeks, I ended up reading two amazing books and being so much more present with my kids. I spent the time I otherwise would have been on the phone making new, healthy habits. It turns out that I was mirroring a study that was done at the University of Pennsylvania, where people were asked to limit their regular use of social media, including Facebook, Instagram, and Snapchat, to no more than thirty minutes a day. After a few weeks, they reported feeling less anxiety, depression, loneliness, and FOMO.

If you're feeling stressed out and overwhelmed, I encourage you to challenge yourself to do the same thing. What habits will you pick up when you're not stuck in the feed? If and when you do go back to using social media, see if you can stay mindful about how using these apps makes you feel. If it's not positive, then it might be time to let 'em go.

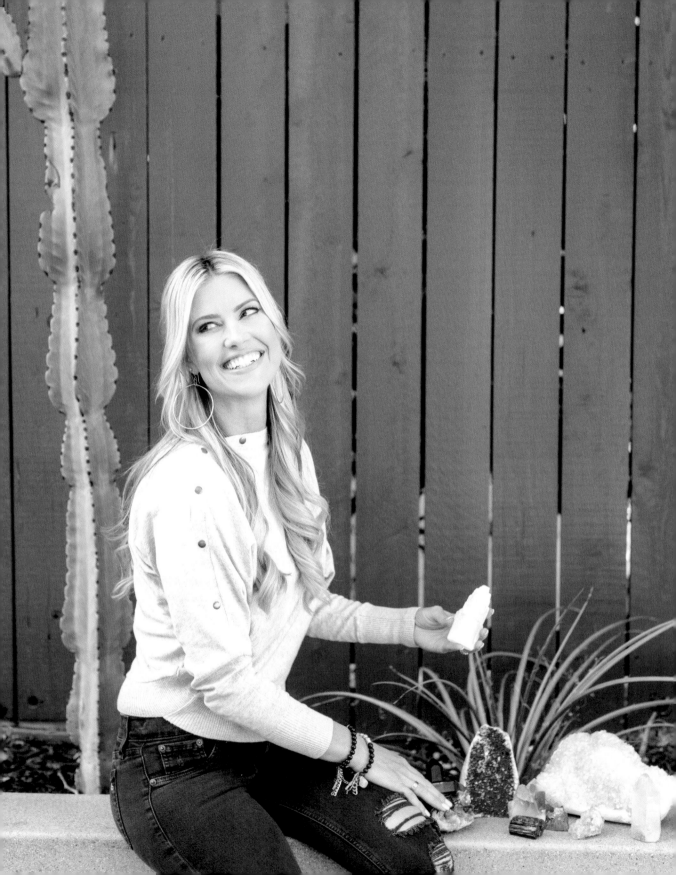

Dream Big

So many of us have a tendency to set goals that are kind of empty or vague, like *Maybe one day I'll get around to this or that.* Part of the reason we're so noncommittal is that we're not truly visualizing what it would look like to make our goals happen. I believe that what we dream and what we visualize has a lot of power—the intentions we set, vocalize, and visualize make an impression in the universe. Taking inventory of what you want for yourself in life and allowing yourself to dream big not only helps you set practical goals but also has a spiritual dimension—it's a way of aligning yourself with your true spirit.

I started this kind of practice when I was in high school. I'd ask myself where I saw my life in five, ten, fifteen years. I'd make lists of the goals I had and things I wanted for myself, from my career to my house to my husband. When I was twenty-two, I hired a real estate coach, and he taught me how to make a vision board. We started with my five-year goals—everything from the places I wanted to visit, to the kids I wanted to have, to the achievements I wanted to accomplish. I would print out pictures that represented these things and pin them up on the board, which was hanging in my office so I could see it every day. And every day I'd be reminded of what I was working toward. Little by little, I got to see these miracles happen as the objects on my board became my reality. Now I have a vision board hanging in my closet, which I update around the New Year. This year my husband and I did ours together on New Year's Eve, which made it that much more special.

To create a vision board, ask yourself where you want to be in five years. Who do you want to be? Who do you want to be with? Have you always wanted to go on safari? Put that on there! Do you want to write a book? Get it on the board! (I did; look at me now!) Have a specific fitness goal? Choose pictures that inspire and motivate you. And give yourself permission to dream BIG. This board is for you and you only—so don't limit yourself because of what other people might think. You can either make a physical board that you keep in your house, or you can make a digital board using an app like Pinterest. Just make sure you're consistently looking at that board. Mine is still in my closet, while Cara keeps hers in her bathroom. That way your goals are present in your mind every day, and both consciously and subconsciously you're moving toward them.

Give Yourself a Time-Out

I'm sure you've *never* experienced this, but you know when your kids are acting all kinds of crazy and aren't listening and barely seem to have any self-control? What's usually the first thing you do? Call a time-out. It might not necessarily be for punishment, but like a mini reset. "Go and sit on the couch and take a breath," or "Go outside and get some fresh air." Right? So why don't we ever do that for ourselves?! We all know when those crazy, overwhelmed, out-of-control feelings are creeping up, yet most of us feel like we just need to power through. Instead, think about parenting your inner child the same way you'd be there for your own children. Give yourself permission to take a break and a breath. You might even say to yourself, "I can tell that you're tired/hungry/upset, and that's okay. Let's do something about that." Take a few minutes to do some breath work, walk around the block, or make yourself a healthy snack. I guarantee that the small amount of time you give yourself will make up for all the time you'd otherwise lose being unable to focus and function.

If you've made it this far, then by now you've done the *work*. You've built the strong foundation by hitting the reset button and learning how to tune in to your body's needs. You've created a fresh new space for yourself as you've gotten your body moving in a gentler, kinder way, and then you let in all that amazing light by nourishing your mind, too. Now there's only one more thing left to do: move in! Turn the key, walk in the door, and inhabit this incredible place. Yes, that means balancing everything you've learned so far with everyday life—kids, work, laundry, car pool, and all. Luckily, as two crazy-busy moms, we've been there. So we've dedicated the next chapter to teaching you how to take these lessons and make them work for you, all day, every day.

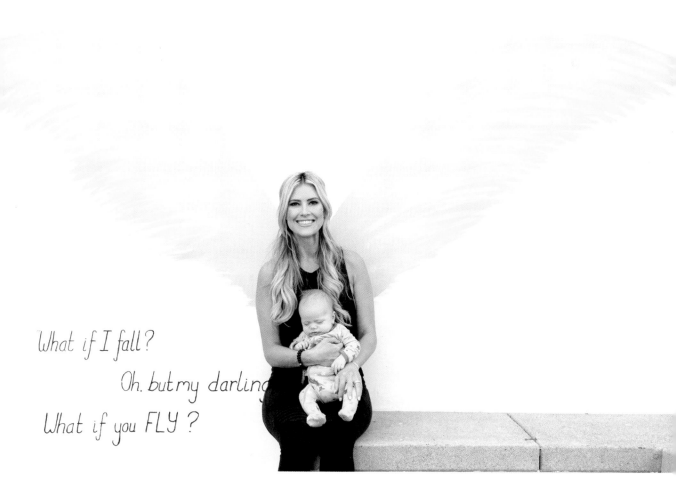

What if I fall?
Oh, but my darling
What if you FLY?

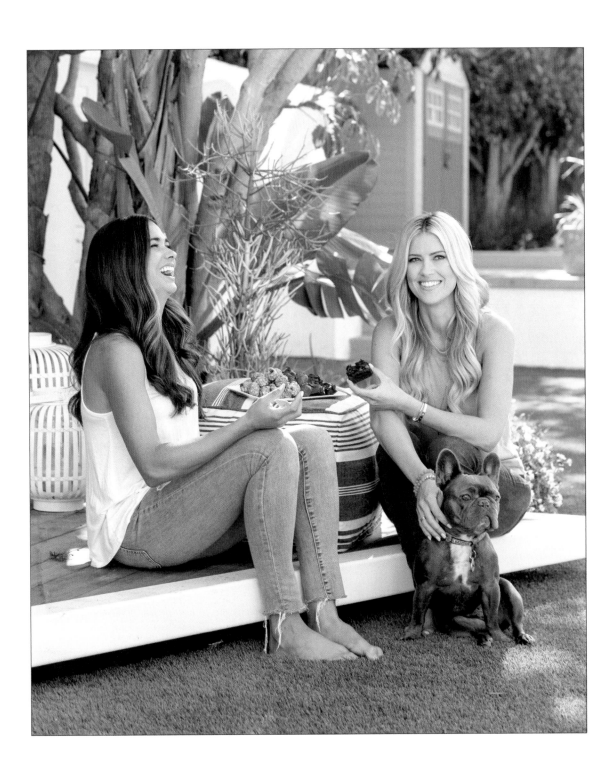

Part IV

MOVING IN

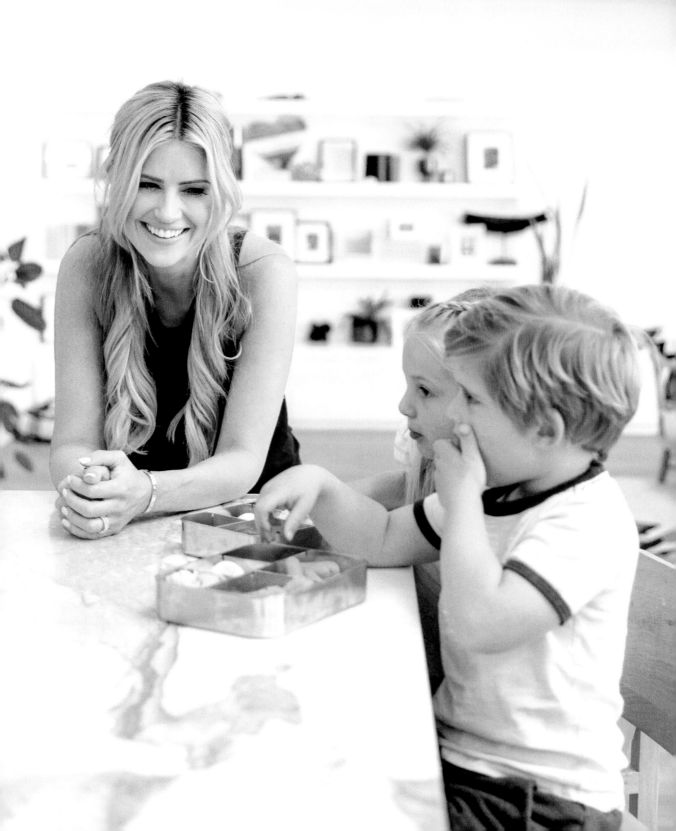

Chapter 8

MAKING IT WORK IN REAL LIFE

Christina: Cara and I are on the same page when it comes to taking care of ourselves. We know just how crucial it is that we do it, but we also live in the real world where it can be hard to make our well-being a priority. It's not like we have all day to spend making beautiful meals, going to yoga, and luxuriating in long baths while we meditate on the meaning of life. That's why anything we do to keep ourselves feeling great and staying sane must fit two criteria: It can't take a lot of time, and it's gotta be something we can do consistently.

To help you figure out how to fold all of your new lessons and tools into your life, we wanted to let you into ours—hot messes and all. There's no such thing as a "perfect day" when the meals are magically made, lunches miraculously packed, and exercise accounted by for 9 AM. Instead, we make it work however we can. A lot of it has to do with embracing the chaos, but we also rely on tons of hacks to stay on top of the things that matter to us most, whether it's having our kitchens stocked with ingredients that can be thrown together for easy meals and snacks (especially if you're less of a planner and more of a fly-by-the-seat-of-your-pants chick like us), prepping meals in advance, time-blocking your to-do list, setting mini goals, and making our workouts work for our lives instead of the other way around.

Here are our favorite remodel hacks that make it possible for us to keep feeling great, no matter what life throws our way.

REMODEL HACK #1
Get Prepared

So many people assume that I'm a planner. I'm organized, for sure, but I've always been a go-with-the-flow kind of girl, and that includes my approach to feeding myself and my kids. I don't always have time to plan out every single meal and snack for the week. I also tend to eat the same foods every week, which helps in the plan-less department. So for me, I like knowing that I have everything I need in the house to make easy meals and snacks throughout the day, plus breakfast for the kids, lunch-packing materials, and what I call free-for-all dinners. This laid-back approach to dinner in our house means there's not a lot of pressure on me to cook every night. On free-for-all nights, everyone gets to have whatever they're in the mood for, because my pantry and fridge are stocked with the building blocks of well-rounded meals.

Cara: I'm like Christina—not much of a meal planner. With four kids and a constantly changing schedule that's built around practices, games, and school activities, even the best-planned week can easily go to pieces. I keep my pantry and fridge full of all the essentials I need for everyone's snacks and meals, including easy no-cook options. Aside from breakfast, which I do like to make in advance and keep stocked in the fridge or freezer (think individually wrapped egg-and-veggie cups, muffins, and sweet potato pancakes that can be quickly warmed up), I want to have lots of flexibility throughout the week for whipping up something nourishing and tasty on the fly.

Our Pantry Staples:

AVOCADOS: Instant snack and super satisfying blended into smoothies, mashed up for dipping veggies, and spread on toast.

BEANS AND LEGUMES: Chickpeas and black beans are Christina's favorites, while Cara has at least four kinds of beans in rotation because they're often a meat stand-in. There's no shame in buying canned instead of dried—they come in handy when the mood strikes for a pot of chili.

BREADS: Whole grain, gluten-free, or both—depending on what works for you and your body.

CHEESE: Christina always has a variety, like mozzarella and goat cheese, plus nondairy options like almond cheese, on hand.

CHICKEN, TURKEY, AND GRASS-FED BEEF: We prefer to buy organic to avoid any hormones or antibiotics that may be have been used when raising the animals. Keep a selection in the freezer and you'll always have a great foundation for dinner, like a stir-fry, soup, or salad.

EGGS: The essential portable protein. Keep a batch of hard-boiled eggs in your fridge to grab as snacks, smash into egg salad, or sprinkle over greens. Eggs take minutes to scramble up in the morning (add a big handful of veggies and a couple slices of avocado you've got yourself a meal!) and are perfect for making ahead in breakfast egg cups or breakfast burritos.

FISH: Wild-caught salmon is in heavy rotation at Christina's house and ends up topping many lunches and dinners.

FLOUR: Cara keeps a stash of almond flour (love the one from Trader Joe's!) and a gluten-free flour blend for all her baking projects.

FRESH AROMATICS: That's fancy talk for onions and garlic. And we buy the pre-chopped versions because who always has the time to mince?!

FRUIT: We keep a variety of frozen fruit for smoothies as well as fresh seasonal fruit. Sticking with seasonal means you'll never get bored and you'll always get the best flavor. Our favorites are bananas, berries, pears, peaches, grapes, and apples. We try to buy organic when we can.

GREEN JUICE: Sometimes it's store- or juice bar–bought because there's not always time to prep a homemade batch, but Christina usually keeps a stash in her fridge so she's sure to get in her five colors a day. Her go-to combo is apples, lemon, cucumber, kale, spinach, carrots, celery, and parsley. Just make sure to enjoy with a protein or fat.

GUACAMOLE, HUMMUS, AND OTHER PREPARED DIPS: Perfect for quick snacks or for dolloping on top of salads. Make sure your hummus is made with no additives and preferably no canola oil. Or, for an even more inexpensive option, make a batch of Cara's favorite hummus (page 211).

KID-FRIENDLY ITEMS: We always have options that can be packed up, like minimally processed chips and crispy things (we love Veggie Straws and Kettle Chips), individual yogurts, applesauce, dried fruit, beef sticks, and a variety of bars (ideally soy-free and low sugar).

KOMBUCHA: Cara loves how this sweet fermented drink improves her digestion. And just like coffee, it's a fun ritual to drink (the bubbles are just like having a soda!). Look for one with no added sugar, preferably organic.

MILK: Almond, coconut, 2 percent—again, whatever works for your body. We both keep a variety on hand and use them for smoothies, overnight oats, and creamy soups.

NUTS: Christina keeps a rotation of nuts in the freezer so she always has a handful nearby for emergency snacking.

NUT BUTTERS: Life-saving as easy snacks (for dipping veggies or fruit), stirred into oats, scooped into smoothies, or eaten by the spoonful. We especially love almond butter and peanut butter.

OATS: What else would you make your overnight oats out of?! Also great served warm, folded into muffins, or tossed into smoothies for the trifecta of carbs, fiber, *and* protein.

OILS AND VINEGARS: Grapeseed oil for cooking and high-quality avocado oil or extra-virgin olive oil for drizzling, plus balsamic vinegar, red and white wine vinegar, brown rice vinegar (great for simple dressings and to add more flavor to a dish without using more salt).

ORGANIC TORTILLA OR RICE CHIPS: For dipping in guacamole and hummus or crumbling into salads or soups.

PASTA: We stock up on a selection of rice, chickpea or legume, and whole wheat pasta for super-quick and easy dinners.

PASTA SAUCE: Simmer with some shredded veggies, add pasta or grains, done.

QUINOA: An all-around go-to, whether it's a base for grain bowls, serving under chicken or fish, tossing into salads, or even making a sweet breakfast porridge.

RICE: Wild, brown, jasmine—mixing it up is always a good idea so you don't get stuck in a flavor or nutrient rut. People are sometimes surprised when we say that we eat jasmine rice, but it has the same nutrient profile and glycemic load as brown!

RICE CAKES: Christina NEVER runs out of these because you don't need more than almond butter and a piece of fruit to make a meal out of them. See if you can find a brown or wild rice version.

SEASONAL VEGGIES: We always have a rotation of fresh veg and lots of it—especially spinach or other leafy greens, mixed greens, carrots, celery, cucumbers, peppers, and sweet potatoes. We also keep a stash in the freezer so we can whip up something with frozen veggies if we've run out of fresh options or we're in the mood for something that's not in season (frozen fruits and veggies are picked at peak seasonality and flash frozen). We are also all about saving time with pre-chopped options!

SEEDS: Hemp, chia, flax—staples for us because they're a great way to add fiber and protein to just about anything.

SPICES AND SEASONINGS: Our essentials are cinnamon, vanilla, sea salt, paprika, and chili powder. If there are other flavors you love, stock up! Dried spices generally stay fresh for up to a year.

SWEETENERS: We choose less-processed sweeteners, especially when baking. Manuka honey or other raw honey is first choice because it has antiviral, anti-inflammatory, and antioxidant benefits. (It's in our first-aid kit, too—it's great for scrapes and sore throats.) Second choice is maple syrup.

UNSWEETENED COCONUT FLAKES: We use these for baking and smoothies.

VEGGIE BURGERS: Cara prefers to not eat beef, so for extra protein variety she keeps these in her freezer. She chooses brands without soy and pea protein and especially loves Hilary's and Dr. Praeger's.

Meal Prep

Even though we just finished telling you that we're not super planners, we do think it's helpful to give some thought to what your week ahead will look like and what recipes or meals might work with your timing or tastes. We totally get that not everyone is going to be comfortable with just winging it, and we

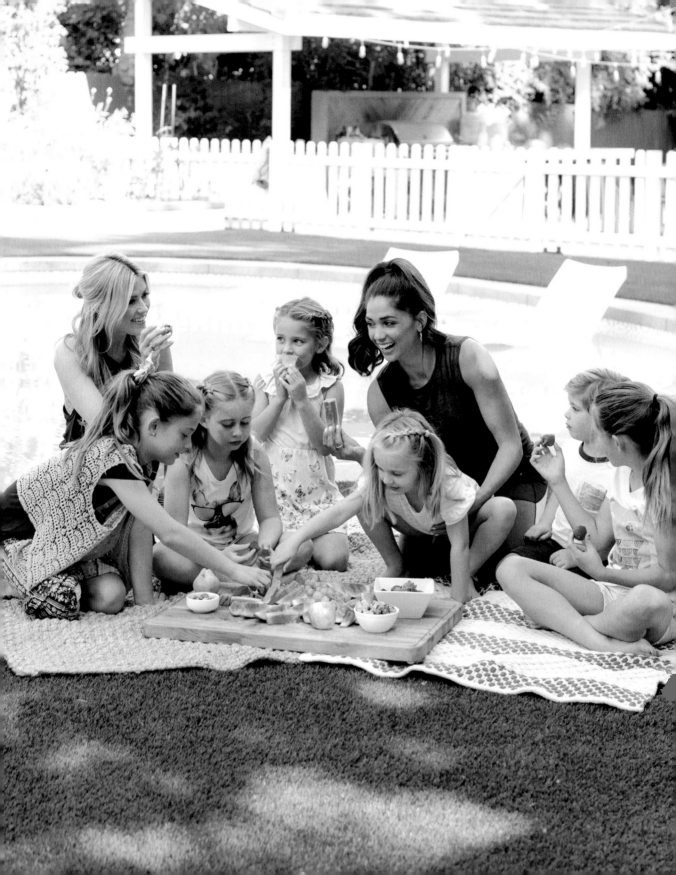

also get that not everyone has the time or desire to come up with a plan and stick with it. So we've come up with our favorite tips and tricks for both the Organized Improviser and the Planner. See which category you fall into and go from there—be honest with yourself! There's no wrong answer, so go with the guidance that best suits you and your life.

FOR THE ORGANIZED IMPROVISER

You fall into this category if you feel more comfortable going with the flow of life than following a set plan. You know that every day is going to throw something crazy at you, and you want to be flexible enough to roll with it. You trust yourself enough to know that even when things get overwhelming you'll still be able to get something nourishing on the table.

- If you don't want to nail down specific dinners for each night of the week but still want to bring some structure and predictability to dinnertime, do what Cara does and come up with a theme like Meatless Mondays, Taco Tuesdays, Stir-Fry Wednesdays, Pasta Thursdays, and Pizza Fridays.
- When you do make dinner, make extra. That way you'll have leftovers to enjoy for lunches or freeze and have for dinner another night.
- Pick two breakfast recipes from chapter 9 each week and prepare double batches over the weekend. Keep the items individually portioned in the fridge or freezer and reheat as needed.
- Prep smoothie ingredients in jars or freezer-safe plastic baggies. All you need to do is dump the ingredients into the blender, add milk, and blend.
- Make a large batch of quinoa or rice for the week and store it in the fridge. Do the same with beans if you buy dried instead of canned.
- Always keep fresh fruit and nuts on hand. It's the ultimate no-recipe recipe for a satisfying no-prep meal! Other easy combos include rice

cakes plus guacamole or nut butter and sliced banana, veggies and hummus or guacamole, and hard-boiled eggs plus fruit.

FOR THE PLANNER

You're a classic type A. You're happiest when you know what to expect and feel most at peace when you have a set plan to reach for when the unexpected happens. When it's time for a meal, you don't want to have to spend the extra time or energy figuring out what to make. You'd much rather do the work in advance and let the little bit of extra time you spent preparing pay off during the busy week.

Select your meals.

- Spend time at the end of each week thinking about the following week (Friday evenings are great for this). Look at your family's schedule and figure out which nights you'll have time to cook versus nights when you'll need to reach for something prepared in advance.
- Write down what you plan to have for breakfast, lunch, dinner, and snacks throughout the week. Use our recipes for inspiration!
- Check your fridge and pantry to see what additional ingredients you'll need. (If you keep up your inventory, you'll see it'll be very few.)

Prep ingredients and make-ahead meals.

- Slice and chop veggies (for snacking or for tossing into salads, eggs, or sautés).
- Assemble mason jar meals, including overnight oats, chia pudding, Greek yogurt parfaits, soup, salads or power bowls (make a few different kinds for the week), or just about any type of leftovers (total game-changer!).

- Make smoothie kits in jars or freezer-safe baggies (everything but the liquid).
- Store premade individually wrapped sandwiches and wraps in the fridge.
- Make a batch of trail mix or granola and store it in snack-sized portions.
- Prepare any recipes that can be stored in the fridge or freezer (most casseroles, slow cooker meals, soups, and stews).

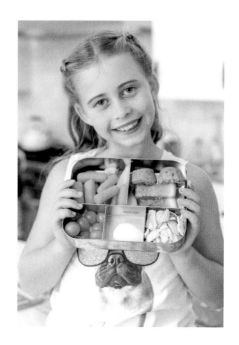

OUR TOP 5 COOKING TIME-SAVERS

1. Buying pre-chopped veggies, especially slaw mixes (more colors and less chopping!).
2. Buying rotisserie chicken, precooked wild shrimp, and premade salmon or ahi tuna burger patties.
3. Doubling or tripling dinner recipes and freezing leftovers (most will be good for up to six months!).
4. Doubling or tripling smoothies and freezing extras in mason jars. Transfer to the fridge the night before you want to enjoy.
5. Making big batches of grains and/or beans and freezing extras (they'll last for four to five months).

Get Your Family Involved

Christina: One of the things I love most about Cara's approach to eating is that it makes sense for every member of the household. As moms, we spend so much time worrying about whether our kids are getting the nutrition they need, but on this program, you don't even have to think twice about it. Not only will their nutritional needs be met, but they will actually eat the food on their plate without complaint—all of the recipes in this book are kid-friendly.

Meal prep is SO much easier when everyone's eating the same thing—no more making separate meals for grown-ups and kids. If my kids knew how many vegetables were on their plates, they'd probably freak out. Cauliflower rice in their tacos? Zucchini in their muffins? Broccoli slaw in their pasta salad? Ew! But not really, because those are some of their favorite and most requested dishes. And when you know that they—like you—are going to get in all their colors (including in their smoothies, granola bites, and brownies!), it's as if a giant weight has been lifted. The transition to eating these new foods as a family may take a little time, but the more your kids see you eating them, the more interested they'll become—a total win-win.

Oh, and if you think that all my kids eat are bell peppers and celery sticks—guess again! Just like the 80/20 rule and enjoying intentioned indulgences are essential parts of the Wellness Remodel plan, that goes for our kids, too. Cara and I both let our kids enjoy themselves at birthday parties or when we all go out for dinner, and we don't sweat it because we know that most of the time, we're giving them food that is going to help them build strong, healthy bodies and feel their best. We also don't make any foods off-limits to them—there's no faster way to make them want a food more than restricting it! I might buy an organic or low-sugar version of a treat my kids want all the time (like root beer), but otherwise it's there for them to have.

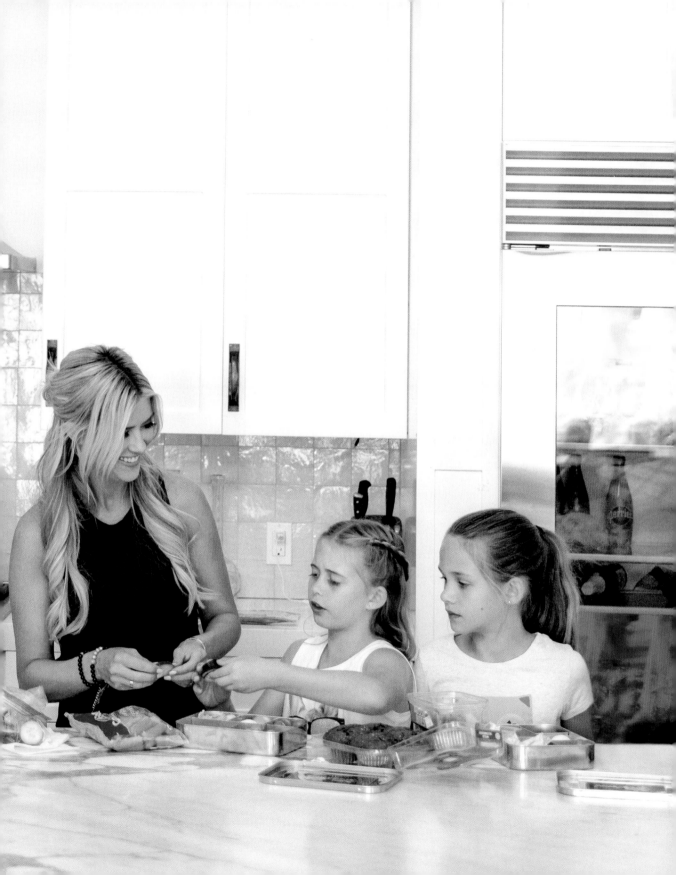

Cara: A very effective way to get your kids involved is to let them help with the decision-making process about what to eat. You'll be there to guide them and make sure they have good choices to choose from, but otherwise, let them take the lead from time to time. Flip through the recipes in this book and see what appeals to them. Let them decide what toppings they're putting on their pizzas or into jars of overnight chia pudding. And if they're old enough (I say five and up), definitely include them in packing their lunches. I love giving my kids bento boxes for school and letting them choose what to put in each section. I provide lots of healthy options—chopped fruit and veggies, hummus, gluten-free chips or other packaged snacks, nuts (if nuts are allowed in their school), dried fruit, granola, cubed cheese, a hard-boiled egg, slices of turkey breast, even repurposed leftovers from the night before. There are also a ton of recipes in chapter 9 that are great for packing up for school (and have lots of veggies secretly tucked inside). The fact that they feel like they have control over these decisions goes a long way in keeping them open-minded about eating foods that nourish them, in addition to trying new ones.

But most important, let your kids know *why* it's important to make these choices. In our house, we're always telling our girls that taking care of their bodies will make them faster and stronger—which means a lot to them because they're budding athletes. They're also learning to listen to their bodies, like being able to tell that eating a fruit rollup for a snack on its own is going to make them feel a little sick. My kids now know that if they're going to eat something carb-y like chips, crackers, pretzels, fruit, or fruit snacks—all the stuff our kids have so much access to—that they should have some string cheese or some nuts or turkey with it. They can *feel* when their bodies are better able to sit and concentrate.

The same thing goes for kids who are struggling with conditions that are affected by diet, such as eczema, allergies, or even ADHD. My daughter Claire gets really itchy if she eats gluten. It's not life or death, but it makes her uncomfortable. So I tell her that she has a choice—she can choose to be comfortable or she can eat the handful of pretzels and deal with the consequences. And sometimes she does! But more often than not, she doesn't. She's beginning to realize that she'd rather avoid the foods that don't make her feel good.

Christina: Don't have kids? You can get your partner, roommate, or even coworkers involved! They may not be following the Wellness Remodel plan, but they can still be supportive if you help them know how. Your partner or roommate can help pick out recipes that you can cook together, or at the very least you can let them know what foods you've decided to leave out of your diet so that they can be respectful when they do the grocery shopping or order in meals. See if your coworkers want to coordinate making lunches and packing snacks for the week. I promise once people start seeing how amazing you look and feel, they'll want to get on the Remodel bandwagon, too. The important thing here is that you find some community to lean on; it'll help make your Remodel experience that much easier and more satisfying.

REMODEL HACK #3
Learn to Be Okay with a Little Chaos

It's inevitable that things won't go the way you planned. Cara and I joke that our lives are like the book *If You Give a Mouse a Cookie*, except it's *If You Give a Mom a Chore*. (Totally going to be our second book!) But seriously, this whole Remodel process is about learning how to live your life while life actually happens. There's no pause button. And no matter how much you pray for it (trust me, I've tried!), there's never going to be a magical day when all you have to do is wake up, go to a yoga class, and drink a smoothie. So you can either totally lose your $*&t, or you can take a deep breath and move on with your life. Or maybe even laugh! Your life AND your health will be so much better for it.

Consider this your official permission to let the small things be small things—leave the dishes in the sink. Rerun the washing machine if you have to. There's always tomorrow! It's okay not to be perfect all the time. Instead, focus on the bigger, more important things that really do bring you healing, energizing joy like spending time with your family, moving your body, and preparing nourishing meals.

That said, Cara and I get that it's not easy for everyone to be more laid-back about a little chaos. So we've put together two of our favorite tools for helping you bless the mess.

Time-Blocking

Cara: Christina sort of does this naturally—mostly out of necessity because she has only a set amount of time between takes—and I saw how efficient it made everything she needed to do in a day. So I took a cue from her and designated set amounts of time for everything on my to-do list. It's a strategy that's really improved my life because I know I'm going to have enough time to do everything I need to do, plus the things I want to do.

HERE'S HOW:

• Start by making your to-do list for the following day. It can be on a scrap of paper, in your e-mail, on a whiteboard—however you like to keep track.

Include everything from chores (laundry, dusting, making beds) to work-related tasks (answering e-mail, finishing assignments) to things like playing with your kids, scouring the Internet for a new yoga mat, and getting in a workout. Put it all on there!

• Now make a schedule. Start with the knowns: how much time you'll need to work, take care of the kids' needs, make meals, work out, etc. Then see how much time is left (no, it's never going to be enough!). Start dedicating set slots for each item you want to accomplish, making sure everything gets at least a little time. Maybe it's twenty minutes for folding the laundry, twenty minutes for answering e-mail three times a day (consolidating e-mail time is another trick I learned from Christina—SO much better than spending all day staring at your in-box!), twenty minutes for loading the dishwasher, one hour for playing outside with the family, and thirty minutes for finally getting to the book club book.

• Get to work! It doesn't matter when in the day or at what hour each task gets done, so long as you're giving each task its assigned amount of time and NO MORE. That's the key—when the fifteen minutes for cleaning up the kitchen are up, move on to the next thing. The important thing is that you don't spend any more time than what's allotted, then check off that item, and move on to the next one.

What you'll come to see is that it's okay if there are still a couple of dishes left in the sink, or a few (non-urgent) e-mails left in your in-box. Guess what? There are always going to be more of those things tomorrow! So why not make sure that you're also spending your time each day doing the things that truly make your life great?

Christina: A lot of the women I meet ask me how I balance having a family and a career. The truth is, no matter how hard I try, I can't always strike the perfect balance between the two. But I can make a choice about the *quality* of the time I spend with my kids and how we connect at home. When I walk in the door, I do my best to be present. My kids' games and activities come first. I'm off my phone, and I'm not thinking about work. I know how much it means to my kids to have my full, uncompromised attention, and it's the very least I can give them. Showing up engaged and ready to follow their lead turns the few hours we have together at night into something meaningful and special. I also try to spend a little time with each of my kids individually so they each feel seen and heard.

Being present with your kids includes taking good care of yourself, too. If you're feeling fuzzy or tired because your food isn't supporting you, or if your head is a mess because you haven't taken the time to just breathe and get centered, then you're not fully there. It's like they tell you in the safety videos on the plane—put on your own oxygen mask before helping small children. The same goes for living a balanced, nourished life.

Setting Daily Mini Goals

Cara: So many of my clients tell me that they don't have time for themselves, and I can totally empathize with that feeling of overwhelm. But I've got news for them (and you): everyone has *some* time to commit to their well-being. If you have ten minutes, then you have plenty. Five? More than enough. Another bad habit that pretty much all of us share is never giving ourselves enough credit or feeling like we never do enough. But I say that something you can accomplish in ten minutes—or five—is still a powerful contribution to your overall wellness.

Some people call these types of exercises micro habits or mini habits because the daily practice ultimately leads you to adopt a new regular practice, and for a longer period of time. But I think that sticking with micro is completely okay, and that starting fresh with your goals each day is a way to stay accountable by constantly asking yourself, "What do I want to accomplish today?"

Here's how it works: Every night, choose one small goal that you will absolutely, no excuses, have time to accomplish the following day. Resist the urge to be an overachiever and pick more than one; that defeats the purpose of setting yourself up for success. Just stick with the one, nail it, and check it off your to-do list for the day (yes, you get to put it on the list AND check it off). Did it feel awesome? Great! Do it again the next day. Or pick something new to try on for size. It's a great way to dip your toe into each of the recommendations in this book, whether it's easing yourself into meditating, working on your burpee reps, or drinking more water. Here are some of our favorite mini habits, all of which take ten minutes or less:

- Do ten minutes of meditation (an app like Meditation Studio has guided meditations, some as short as five minutes).
- Do 20 push-ups and 20 squats (Cara loves this one so she can check off "exercise" from her list no matter what!).
- Make a smoothie.
- Read for ten minutes (doesn't matter what it is! Our minds need the time to focus on something we enjoy).
- Get in 10,000 steps (sounds like a lot, but it's really not!).
- Take a multivitamin and probiotic.
- Drink 80 ounces of water (over the course of the day, not all at once!).

- Share a quote that makes you happy.
- Offer gratitude for three things before your feet hit the ground in the morning.
- Add an item to your vision board.

Fit in Your Daily Activity during Everyday Life

Even as someone who encourages people to move more for a living, I'll be the first to say that sometimes getting in a consistent workout routine can be hard! Especially if you have young kids or an unpredictable work schedule. There was a time in my life when I would exercise at the same time every day, rain or shine, and get frustrated if it didn't happen. But after years of having kids, life has reminded me that I don't always get to call the shots; I've learned to go with the flow. And I'm happier and less stressed out because of it.

So instead of a rigid workout schedule that I stuck to in order to optimize what my body looked like, now I work out any hour of the day I can squeeze it in, and I do it just to get my heart rate going and boost my serotonin levels. Because I know how important those factors are to my health, it makes it easier to hold myself accountable—even if means including the kids in a workout or getting in thirty minutes of activity after they go to bed. To keep myself motivated, I make a deal with myself that no matter what, I'm going to get to one of my favorite group classes at least once a week. I'm usually so happy that I get to sneak away for an hour that it makes the other three to four workouts I get in the rest of the week seem less like a chore and more like a special treat.

Make Working Out Work for You

In reality, the less time we have for ourselves, the more we need our workouts. So break out of crazy work schedules and family obligations and make it fun for everyone! Here are some effective and fun workout ideas for when you're short on time or need to involve the whole family:

• GO ONLINE: Between Pinterest, YouTube, Facebook, and Instagram, there is no shortage of twenty- or thirty-minute workouts available online. Search for "body weight workouts" or "HIIT workouts."

• SET UP SOCCER AND/OR BASKETBALL DRILLS: Set up drills for your kids and then get in on the action. Include things like high knees or pretend jump rope. Just keep moving for thirty minutes! This is a major double-win if your kids are at the age where they're starting to play competitive sports.

• JUMP ON A TRAMPOLINE: Trampolines for adult workouts (called rebounders) have become all the rage in the wellness world because they help you get all the benefits of jogging but without the high impact. I have clients who have purchased a rebounder for themselves and then taken turns bouncing with their kids. If your family has a big trampoline in the backyard, chase your kids in circles, or play our favorite game, Rocket, where your kids sit in the middle and you see how high you can bounce them. Another (deceptively hard) challenge is to see who can do a trick the highest number of times in a row without messing up. I once did this with plank touches and got to fifty. I was so sore the next day!

• GO OLD-SCHOOL: Play tag or kickball with your kids! They will want to play forever, and it's always good for some laughs (and a sweat).

• SQUAT CLEANUP: Usually cleaning up around the house is a chore, but I say make the most of it and turn it into a workout. Hit a deep squat as you pick up each item on the floor and challenge yourself to see how many you can do. I've gotten to five hundred squats before, thanks to a few different sets of blocks and Legos.

• PLANK-WALK CLEANUP: A variation on the above. Set up in a plank and walk on your hands and feet to each piece of laundry/dog toy/children's toy, then to the appropriate bin. Harder than it sounds!

Your New-Normal Life Checklist

To help you put all these pieces together and fit them into your normal (but new-and-improved) life, we came up with this handy checklist. Even if you're not a planner, taking five minutes to go through these items before each new week and each new day is a powerful way to keep yourself moving in a direction that's in line with your goals. After these new habits start to take root, coming back to this list on a regular basis will ensure that you're continuing to grow and flourish.

BEFORE THE NEW WEEK:
• Meal plan and prep (washing and slicing veggies, batch-cooking grains, cooking/baking make-ahead meals).
• Set two new goals for the week (being more present during your nighttime routine with the kids, starting one new mindfulness practice, cooking one more meal at home, etc.).
• Schedule your workouts. Look at the week ahead and choose which days you'll commit to exercising for at least thirty minutes.

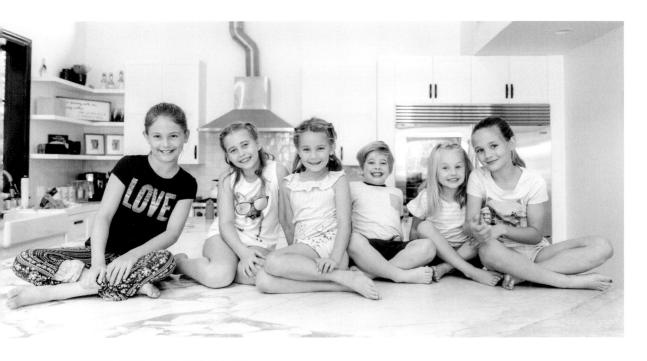

BEFORE EACH NEW DAY:

- Prep meals and snacks; pack up anything that might be necessary on the go.
- Game plan when you'll take a moment to enjoy your meals and snacks throughout the day.
- If it's a designated workout day, find one thirty-minute window. Otherwise, think about how you can integrate more movement into other moments of your day—could you stretch during soccer practice? Challenge your kids to a game of after-school tag?
- Find one ten-minute window for mindfulness of choice (stretching, breathing, journaling, meditating).
- Choose (and commit to!) your phone-down, lights-dimmed, jammies-on, butt-in-bed, wind-down time (ideally one hour before you go to bed, which would ideally be seven to nine hours before you'll wake up).

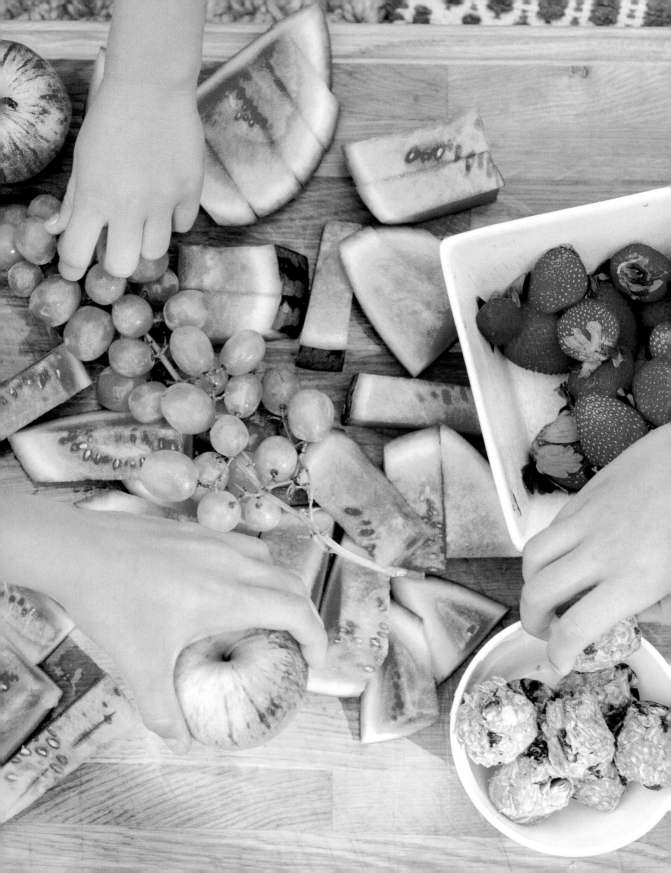

Chapter 9

RECIPES

We were almost hesitant to call this chapter "recipes" because for some people that word brings to mind dishes that are complicated, require a ton of new ingredients, and involve way too much time and energy to plan for and prepare. But this book is all about serving up realness, and these recipes are no exception. They are the time-tested, gold-starred, kid-requested staples that we go back to over and over again. Most of them can be made from what you're already going to be keeping in your pantry (or can be customized so that they do), call for a small handful of ingredients, and take very little time (and skill) to throw together.

These recipes are your greatest allies for make-ahead meals, weeknight family dinners, and portable snacks. But while these dishes are functional and practical, there's nothing boring or utilitarian about them. From the almost-too-indulgent-to-be-breakfast Choco Maca Chia Pudding; to Christina's go-to on-set lunch, the Loaded Deli Sandwich; to the always-in-our-purse Baked Oatmeal Bars; to the kid- and adult-pleasing Coconut Shrimp Tacos with Mango Salsa and Avocado Cilantro Sauce; to Dark Chocolate Sea Salt Freezer Fudge (a Cara-approved dessert AND snack—does it get better than that?!); and Pomegranate Spritzers for when we need to let loose, these recipes are all about living life and making it more delicious.

So make them work for you! Don't be afraid of ingredient swaps and exchanges. Eat breakfast for lunch or dinner for breakfast. Or do what Christina does and eat the same darn thing almost every day! Because each of these recipes follows Cara's plan to a T, all you have to do is listen to what your body really wants and then give it what it needs. Bon appétit!

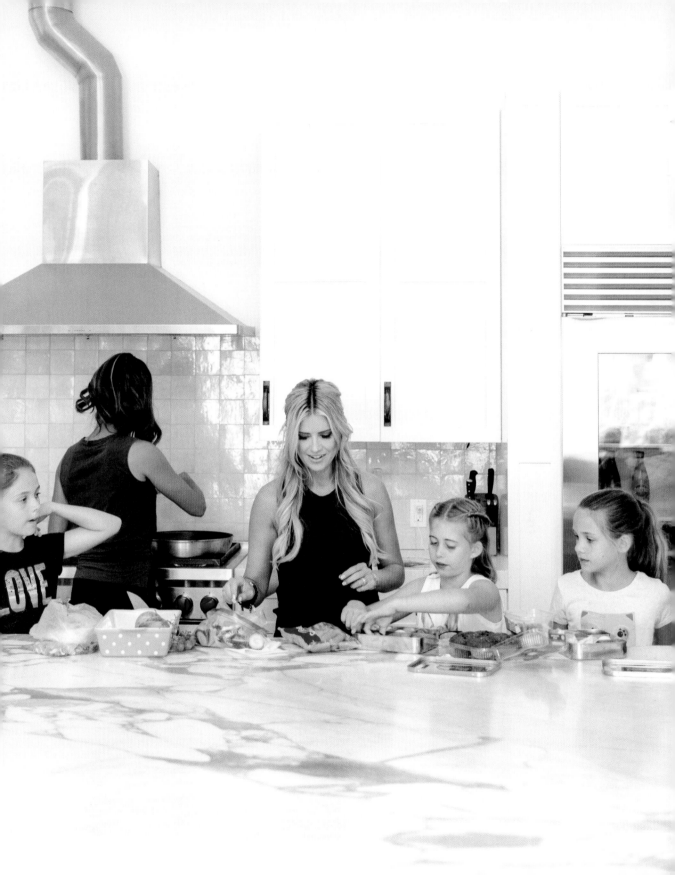

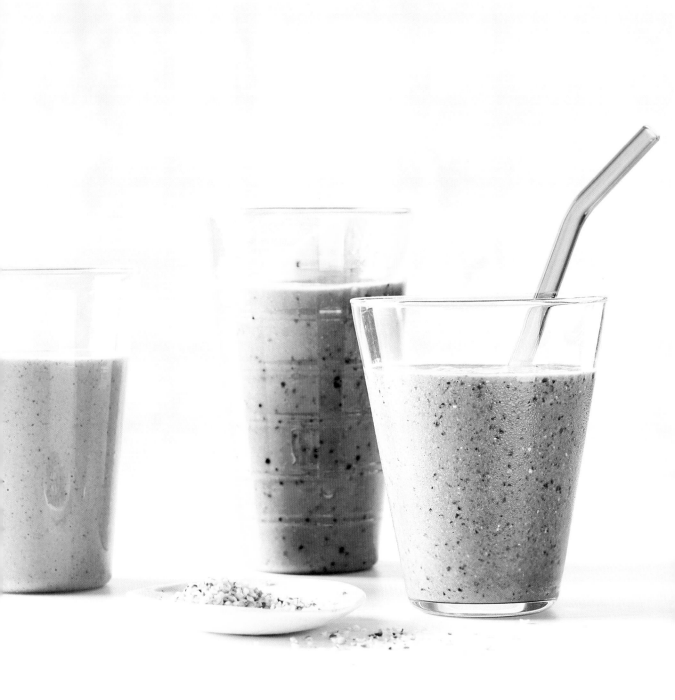

Breakfast

BANANA-VANILLA-FIG SMOOTHIE

We love this smoothie because it finally gives us a reason to use the dried figs we always see at the grocery store. Figs give this blend a hint of sweetness that teams up with the banana, vanilla, and cardamom for a breakfast that's good enough to serve for dessert!

Makes 1 smoothie

Big handful of greens

1 frozen banana, broken in half

4 fresh or dried figs, stemmed

¼ cup raw cashews (soaked in ½ cup filtered water overnight and drained)

1 tablespoon hemp hearts

½ teaspoon pure vanilla extract

Pinch of ground ginger

Pinch of ground cardamom

1 cup unsweetened almond milk

Ice (optional)

Combine all of the ingredients in a blender and blend until smooth.

LEMON-GINGER DETOX SMOOTHIE

There's something so satisfying and empowering when the foods you choose to eat are actively working toward detoxification. This smoothie is amazing to that end because lemon, ginger, and turmeric are all ideal ingredients for encouraging your body to not only let go of damaging toxins but also heal any inflammation. Black pepper may seem like a strange ingredient for a smoothie, but it delivers health-protecting phytochemicals while it also helps to activate the healing power of turmeric. Turmeric needs black pepper like a Q needs a U!

Makes 1 smoothie

1 frozen banana, broken in half

Large handful of spinach

¼ cup plus 2 tablespoons
   almond milk

¼ cup cashews (soaked in ½ cup
   filtered water overnight and
   drained)

¼ cup shredded carrots
   (or 6 baby carrots)

Juice of 1 small lemon

1 tablespoon flax meal

Zest of ½ small lemon

½-inch slice fresh ginger root
   or ¼ teaspoon ground ginger
   (or more, to taste)

¼ teaspoon ground turmeric

Sprinkle of freshly ground
   black pepper

Ice (optional)

Combine all of the ingredients in a blender and blend until smooth.

CINNAMON-PEAR SMOOTHIE

In addition to being juicy and sweet, pears are loaded with pre-biotic fiber, which not only helps your body soak up all the nutrients it needs from your food, but it also keeps you feeling more satisfied after a meal. This smoothie will help power you through the morning and fend off hunger pangs.

Makes 1 smoothie

Big handful of greens
½ frozen banana
1 medium pear, cored, seeded, and
  chopped

2 tablespoons unsweetened
  almond butter
½ cup unsweetened almond milk
1 teaspoon ground cinnamon
Ice (optional)

Combine all of the ingredients in a blender and blend until smooth.

CHERRY-BERRY PIE SMOOTHIE

One of the really fun things about smoothies is that they combine the flavors and textures of the foods that you love but that don't necessarily love you back. This smoothie scratches the itch for cherry pie, complete with the sweet jammy filling (cherries and berries) and dense, buttery crust (almond butter and oats). Do yourself a favor and give yourself time to sit down and eat this one with a spoon!

Makes 1 smoothie

Big handful of greens

½ cup frozen cherries

½ cup mixed berries

2 tablespoons rolled oats

1 tablespoon unsweetened
  almond butter

1 teaspoon pure vanilla extract

1 tablespoon chia seeds
  (optional)

1 cup unsweetened almond milk or
  coconut milk

Ice (optional)

Combine all of the ingredients in a blender and blend until smooth.

GREEN MANGO BLAST SMOOTHIE

Mango is a smoothie secret weapon. First, it makes smoothies creamy and rich (the only way they should be!). Second, it's the perfect amount of sweet. And third, it contains digestive enzymes, which help break down starchy foods. Basically, you can't go wrong by adding mango, especially when you combine it with celery and spinach.

Makes 1 smoothie

2 large handfuls of baby spinach

1 cup frozen mango chunks, plus more for serving

2 stalks of celery

½ cup coconut or nut milk

¼ cup cashews (soaked in ½ cup filtered water overnight and drained)

1 tablespoon hemp hearts

Squeeze of fresh lemon juice

Ice (optional)

Combine all of the ingredients in a blender and blend until smooth. Top your smoothie with additional mango, if desired.

COCONUT-PISTACHIO CHIA PUDDING

We love chia pudding because it can be made the night before and grabbed on the way out the door the next morning. This pistachio-coconut combo is to die for!

Serves 2

1 cup unsweetened coconut milk

¼ cup chia seeds

¼ teaspoon pure vanilla extract

1 teaspoon pure maple syrup or raw honey (optional)

2 tablespoons unsalted shelled pistachios (soaked overnight in filtered water, if possible)

2 tablespoons unsweetened shredded coconut

In a medium bowl, stir together the coconut milk, chia seeds, vanilla, and maple syrup or honey, if using. Cover, transfer to the fridge, and let the chia set overnight. Divide between two jars and top each with 1 tablespoon of the pistachios and coconut.

CHOCO MACA CHIA PUDDING

Maca is a superfood that is known to boost energy, stabilize hormones, and benefit mood. It has a subtle sweet taste that pairs perfectly with chocolatey cacao powder.

Serves 2

1 cup unsweetened coconut milk or nut milk

3 pitted dried dates

3 tablespoons chia seeds

3 tablespoons unsweetened almond butter (or other nut/seed butter)

2 tablespoons cacao powder

2 teaspoons maca powder

Pinch of sea salt

Optional toppings: cacao nibs berries, unsweetened coconut flakes, chopped nuts

Combine all of the ingredieants in a blender and blend on high speed until smooth. Divide the mixture between two jars and refrigerate for at least 2 hours or overnight. Top as desired and enjoy.

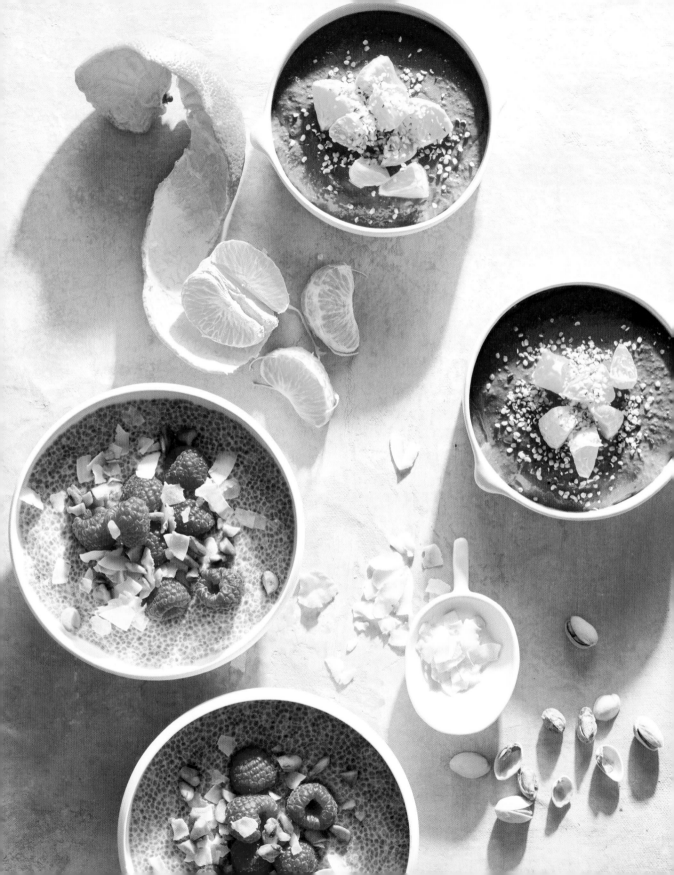

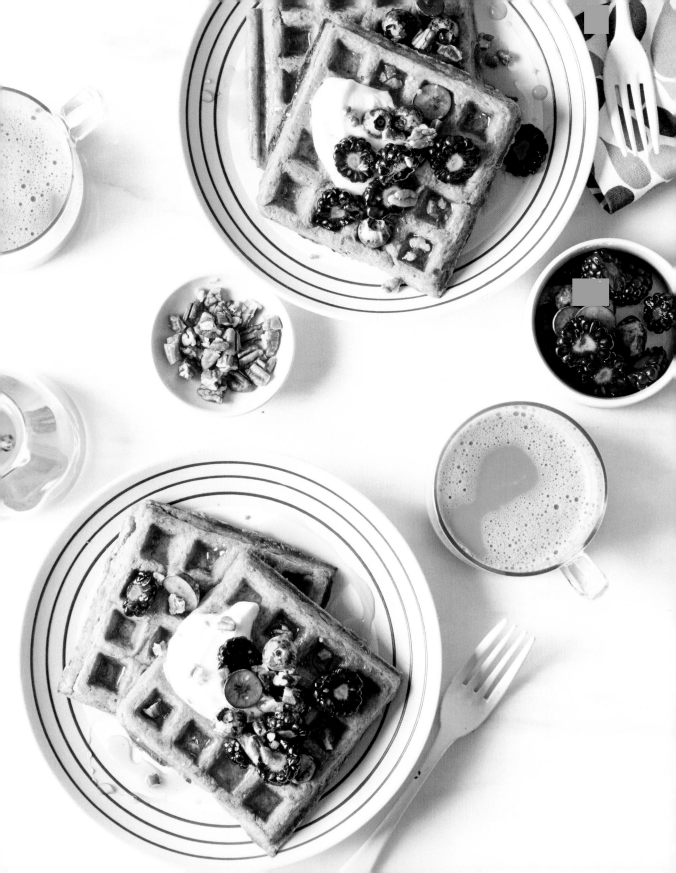

SWEET POTATO AND PECAN WAFFLES

This is a perfect breakfast for those mornings when you want to slow down a little and make a nice, hot meal. And because you can easily freeze these waffles and pop 'em in the toaster to reheat, they're also great for mornings that aren't slow! Our kids love these waffles, which get a bright orange color from the sweet potatoes.

Serves 4

- 1 medium sweet potato, baked until tender, skin removed, and mashed (about ¾ cup)
- 1 cup rolled oats
- 1 cup unsweetened almond, coconut, or cashew milk
- 2 eggs or egg replacer equivalent
- 3 tablespoons unsweetened almond butter
- 1 tablespoon flax meal
- 2 teaspoons baking powder
- 1 teaspoon pure vanilla extract
- 1 teaspoon ground cinnamon
- Zest of 1 medium clementine
- Pinch of ground cardamom
- Pinch of ground nutmeg
- ½ cup chopped pecans, plus more for topping
- Olive oil cooking spray
- Maple syrup, for serving (optional)

Combine all of the ingredients except the pecans in a blender or food processor and blend until relatively smooth (there may still be some lumps; that's okay). Fold in the pecans.

Preheat a waffle iron to medium heat and grease with cooking spray. Pour about ¾ cup of the batter into the center of the waffle iron. Press closed and cook until the waffle is golden brown and the edges are slightly crisp, 3 to 4 minutes. Flip and repeat on the other side. Serve warm topped with pecans and a drizzle of maple syrup, if desired.

PUMPKIN-PECAN PANCAKES

This recipe puts to use two ingredients that have been on the no-no list for far too long: whole wheat flour and yogurt. If after performing a detox you've determined that gluten and/or dairy don't disagree with your system, then feel free to enjoy! (Otherwise, just substitute a gluten-free flour blend and nondairy yogurt.) Either way, you still get to reap all the antioxidant and fiber benefits of pumpkin.

Serves 4 to 6

1 cup whole wheat flour or almond flour

1 tablespoon chia seeds

1 teaspoon pumpkin pie spice

1 teaspoon baking powder

1/2 teaspoon baking soda

Pinch of salt

¾ cup pumpkin puree (NOT pumpkin pie filling)

⅔ cup unsweetened almond, coconut, or cashew milk

½ cup 2 percent plain Greek yogurt or nondairy yogurt

2 tablespoons pure maple syrup (optional), plus more for serving

1 large egg or egg replacer equivalent

1 tablespoon coconut oil

½ cup chopped pecans (optional), plus more for serving

In a medium bowl, whisk together the flour, chia seeds, pumpkin pie spice, baking powder, baking soda, and salt. Set aside.

In a large bowl, whisk together the pumpkin puree, milk, yogurt, maple syrup, egg or egg replacer, and oil. Slowly add the dry ingredients into the mixture and whisk until well combined. Gently fold in the pecans.

Heat a griddle or large skillet over medium heat. Pour the batter on the preheated griddle or pan ¼ cupful at a time. Cook until bubbles appear on the surface of the batter and the edges are lightly browned, 3 to 4 minutes. Flip the pancakes and repeat. Enjoy warm with your favorite toppings.

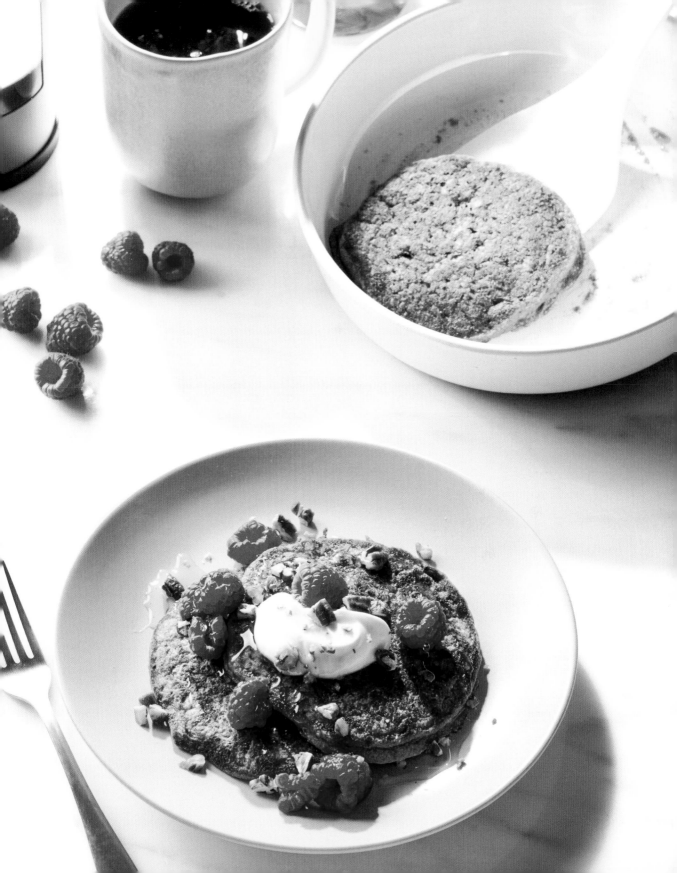

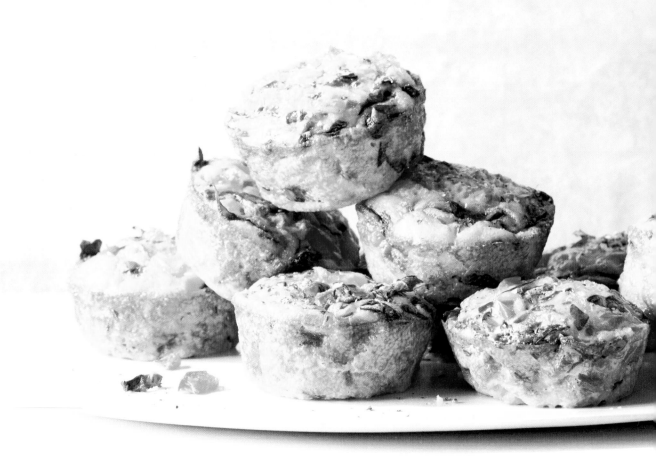

HEARTY VEGGIE EGG CUPS

These bites are bursting with all the good-for-you colors you need to start your day on the right foot, plus a healthy dose of protein and carbs (the rice makes these super satisfying). Make them in advance, store in the freezer, then pop in the oven or microwave in the morning for a grab-and-go breakfast that gives you the fuel you need to conquer your morning.

Serves 4

Coconut oil cooking spray

8 large eggs

2 cups chopped of any of the
   following:

   Kale (chopped)

   Baby spinach (finely chopped)

   Broccoli (chopped)

   Onions (finely chopped)

   Red bell peppers (finely chopped)

   Green bell peppers
      (finely chopped)

   Mushrooms (finely chopped)

1 tablespoon finely chopped
   fresh basil

1 cup cooked wild or brown rice

Kosher salt and freshly ground
   black pepper

Preheat the oven to 350°F. Spray a nonstick muffin tin with cooking spray and set aside.

In a large bowl, whisk the eggs. Add your veggies of choice, the basil, and rice and season with salt and pepper. Divide the egg mixture among the muffin wells, leaving ¼ inch at the top. Bake for 20 minutes, or until a toothpick or knife inserted in the center of a muffin comes out clean. Run a knife around the edges of the muffins to release them from the pan and let them cool.

Store the muffins in an airtight container in the fridge for up to 6 days, or freeze for up to 1 month.

BREAKFAST PIZZA

We usually save this "pizza" for special occasions, because we don't indulge in gluten and dairy every day, but you could swap in cauliflower crust and use nondairy cheese to make this a part of your weekly rotation. We typically whisk the eggs together, but you can also just crack them right on top of the flatbread and then bake them for a crowd-pleasing sunny-side-up option, perfect for wowing your brunch guests.

Serves 4

½ cup shredded mozzarella cheese

4 pieces whole grain naan or flatbread, or 1 cauliflower crust

1 cup baby spinach

1 small tomato, sliced

1 tablespoon sliced green onions (white and green parts)

4 large eggs, whisked

1 avocado, sliced

Preheat the oven to 450°F.

Divide the cheese evenly among the flatbreads. Top with the spinach, tomato, green onions, and eggs. Bake for 25 minutes, or until the eggs are cooked, the cheese has melted, and the vegetables have softened.

Arrange the avocado slices over each pizza, then cut into slices and serve.

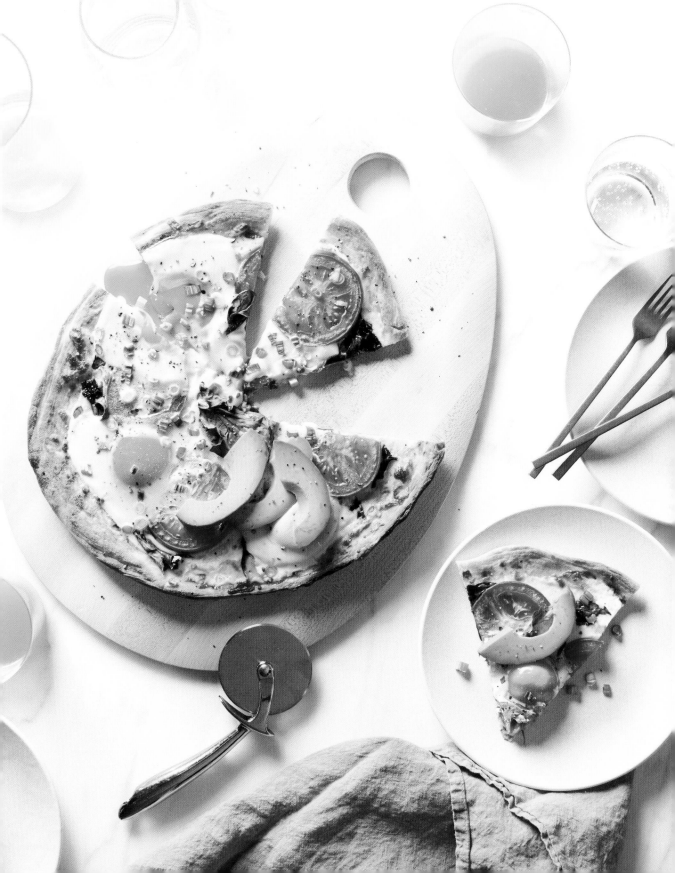

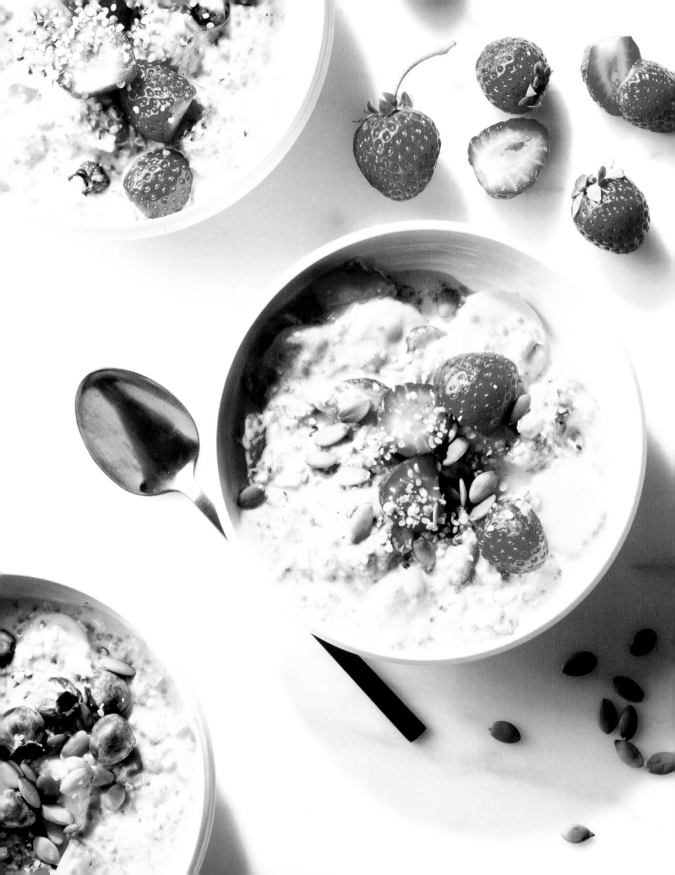

PB&J OVERNIGHT OATS

Peanut butter sometimes gets a bad rap now that other nut butters are widely available, but it is a great source of protein and fat, and unless you are highly sensitive or allergic, there is nothing wrong with enjoying a healthy spoonful. These overnight oats are pretty much the Christina Anstead special. She loves this recipe because it takes minutes to toss together and is super easy to eat on the road—not to mention, it tastes like a grown-up version of PB&J!

Serves 1

½ cup rolled oats

1 tablespoon chia seeds

½ teaspoon ground cinnamon

½ teaspoon pure vanilla extract

½ cup berries (strawberries, blueberries, raspberries, etc.)

½ banana, sliced

1 tablespoon unsweetened peanut butter (or almond butter)

1 cup unsweetened almond milk

In a pint-sized jar, combine the oats, chia seeds, cinnamon, and vanilla and mix well. Add the berries, banana, and peanut butter and pour the milk over the top. Close up the jar and store in the fridge to eat in the morning. Enjoy cold or warm.

FIVE REASONS TO EAT BREAKFAST EVERY DAY

Cara: In my job, I hear "I'm not a breakfast person" a lot. And I get it—I didn't always live for breakfast the way I do now. Like so many of you, I preferred sleep and set aside minimal time to provide myself with the metabolic booster that breakfast contributes to our system. At some point after college, I realized that maybe the reason my body didn't burn fat properly was because my coffee wasn't cutting it as a breakfast option. Once I started studying nutrition, I learned more about what I had been depriving myself of. As you now know, restricting calories is not the way to go, especially first thing in the morning. If anything, it's the best time of day to indulge. And now, with my own family, we try to sit down to breakfast as much as possible, even with the early school schedules. I ask the girls what they want every morning and work with their suggestions and of course their "help." It's probably the only meal of the day I get to sit down and eat mindfully with the kids—like the calm before the storm.

If you're one of those non-breakfast people, hopefully these reasons to eat in the morning will change your mind!

IT BREAKS THE FAST. While you sleep, your body is in a fasting state and your blood sugar is stable. But once you wake up, it's important to let your blood sugar know that you're awake—ideally, by eating within an hour of getting up. The only exception is if you're working out right away; you can wait until after, if you prefer.

IT LOWERS YOUR CHANCES OF OBESITY. Consistently providing your body with fuel throughout the day prevents the end-of-day binging that leads to fat storage. This in turn lowers your risk of heart disease.

IT REVS YOUR SYSTEM. Not only does eating first thing in the morning prevent fat storage, but it also speeds up your metabolism and allows your system to burn at a faster rate.

IT GIVES YOU ENERGY. Eating breakfast fuels your muscles and cells, and it boosts mental clarity, too.

IT'S FUN! I've yet to meet someone who doesn't love a great breakfast. It's easy to get creative with quick breakfasts or create a more indulgent traditional spread with a healthy twist.

GOOD MORNING MUFFINS

*Sometimes you just want a baked treat in the morning, but ide-
ally one that won't send your blood sugar crashing before lunch.
With plenty of protein and a serving of both fruit and vegetables,
these muffins will do the trick. Like any good recipe, this one is
also highly adaptable: You can change up the dried fruit or fold
in any kind of shredded vegetable or nut/seed butter that you like.*

Makes 15 muffins

Coconut oil, for greasing (if not using
   muffin cups)

1 large banana

½ cup rolled oats

⅓ cup unsweetened cashew butter

3 eggs or egg replacer equivalent

¼ cup packed pitted dates

2 tablespoons raw honey or pure
   maple syrup (optional)

2 tablespoons flax meal

2 tablespoons hemp seeds

1 teaspoon baking soda

1 teaspoon pure vanilla extract

1 teaspoon ground cinnamon

½ teaspoon ground ginger

¼ teaspoon ground cardamom

½ teaspoon sea salt

2 large carrots, peeled and
   shredded

1 medium apple (I like Granny
   Smith or Braeburn), peeled, cored,
   and diced

⅓ cup unsweetened dried fruit
   of your choice (such as raisins,
   blueberries, cherries, or currants)

⅓ cup chopped walnuts, pecans,
   or a nut mix

Preheat the oven to 375°F. Line 15 wells of a muffin tin with muffin cups
or lightly grease with coconut oil and set aside.

In a blender, combine the banana, oats, cashew butter, eggs or egg
replacer, dates, honey or maple syrup (if using), flax meal, hemp seeds,
baking soda, vanilla, cinnamon, ginger, cardamom, and salt. Pulse until
the mixture is smooth. Transfer the mixture to a large bowl and gently
fold in the carrots, apple, dried fruit, and nuts until well mixed.

(cont.)

Divide the batter evenly among the muffin cups, filling them about three-quarters full. Bake until the tops of the muffins are golden brown and a toothpick or knife inserted in the center comes out clean, 15 to 20 minutes. Allow the muffins to cool for at least 10 minutes, then transfer them to a wire rack to cool completely.

Store the muffins in an airtight container at room temperature for up to 1 week, in the fridge for about 2 weeks, or in the freezer for up to 1 month.

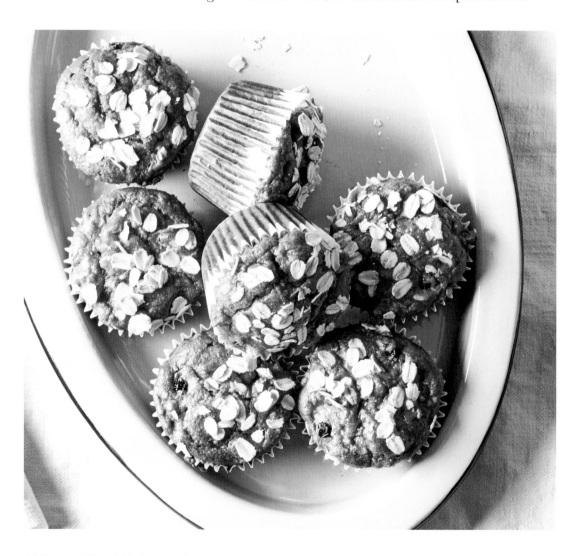

Snacks

HARVEST OAT MUFFINS

Christina is always looking for new recipes for muffins, brownies, and bars—things she can take with her as snacks but will also scratch the itch for something sweet. The best thing about these oat muffins—aside from being delicious—is that they also pack a sizable amount of plant-based nutrition (just be sure you're buying products that include only the pureed apple and pumpkin and not any added sugars!). These muffins can be stored in the fridge for quick bites during the day, and can be frozen and thawed at room temperature the night before you want to enjoy them.

Makes 16 muffins

Olive oil cooking spray

1 cup pumpkin puree (NOT pumpkin pie filling)

½ cup unsweetened applesauce

½ cup pure maple syrup

2 large eggs, beaten

½ teaspoon pure vanilla extract

1 cup rolled oats

½ cup almond flour

2 tablespoons flax meal

1½ teaspoons pumpkin pie spice

1 teaspoon baking soda

½ teaspoon sea salt

1 medium sweet/tart apple (such as Golden Delicious, Honeycrisp, or Pink Lady), peeled, cored, and chopped

½ cup chopped pecans

2 tablespoons pepitas

(cont.)

203

Preheat the oven to 375°F. Lightly grease a 16-well muffin tin or silicone baking cups with cooking spray and set aside.

In a large bowl, combine the pumpkin puree, applesauce, maple syrup, eggs, and vanilla. Mix well.

In a second large bowl, combine the oats, flour, flax meal, pumpkin pie spice, baking soda, and salt. Mix well.

Working slowly, add the dry ingredients to the wet and mix until fully combined. The batter will be a little lumpy—don't overmix! Gently fold in the chopped apple, pecans, and pepitas. Divide the batter among the prepared muffin cups and bake for 30 to 35 minutes, until the muffins are golden brown around the edges and a toothpick or knife inserted in the center comes out clean. Let them cool for about 10 minutes before transferring to a wire rack to cool completely. Store in the fridge for up to 1 week or in the freezer for up to 1 month.

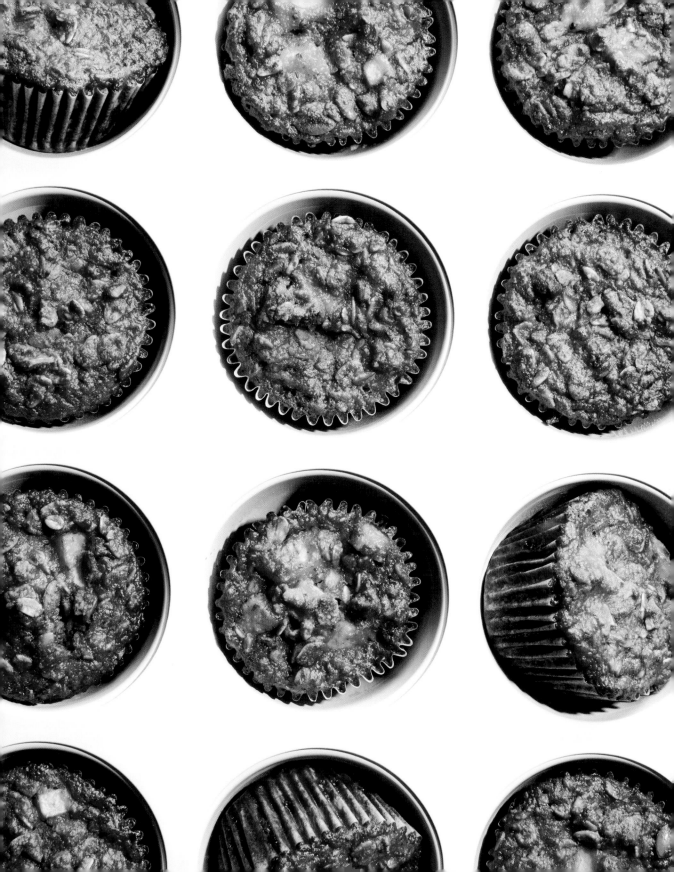

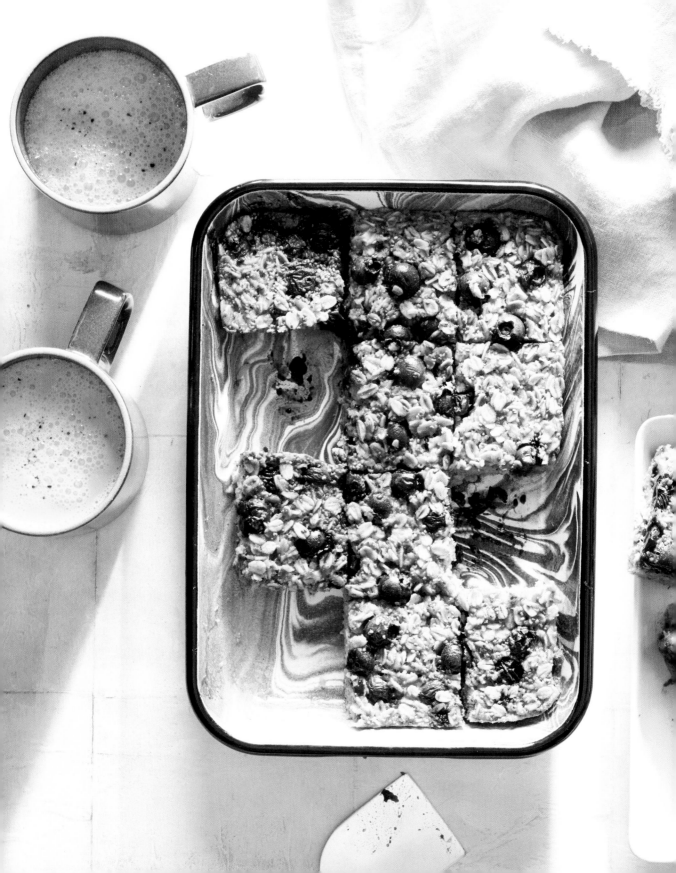

BAKED OATMEAL BARS

These snacks are a special treat for adults and kids alike. Yes, they contain some sugar in the form of maple syrup and bananas, but they're also loaded with fiber and protein and balanced with fat, in addition to collagen peptides, a source of protein that supports gut health and strengthens your bones, joints, hair, and nails (though you could also use a vegan protein powder). Slice these up and individually wrap them for snacks.

Makes about 12 bars

Coconut oil or coconut oil
  cooking spray

2 cups rolled oats

2 scoops collagen peptides (or
  vegan pea protein)

2 tablespoons chia seeds

1 teaspoon baking powder

1 teaspoon ground cinnamon

½ teaspoon kosher salt

2 cups unsweetened
  almond milk

1 ripe banana, mashed

⅓ cup maple syrup

1 large egg

1 teaspoon pure vanilla extract

1½ cups blueberries

Preheat the oven to 350°F. Grease a 10-inch casserole dish with coconut oil or cooking spray and set aside.

In a large bowl, combine the oats, collagen peptides, chia seeds, baking powder, cinnamon, and salt.

In another large bowl, mix together the almond milk, banana, maple syrup, egg, and vanilla. Add the wet ingredients to the dry and mix to combine. Gently fold in the blueberries.

Pour the mixture into the prepared casserole dish to create an even layer. Bake for 30 minutes, or until the edges are golden and the middle has set. Allow the baked oatmeal to cool for 10 minutes, then slice into roughly 2-inch x 2-inch squares. Cool completely and store in a covered container in the fridge for up to 5 days.

CRAVING CRUSHER GRANOLA

It's always a good idea to have nuts, trail mix, or granola on hand for when we need to sneak in a snack but don't have time to prep anything in advance. While this version of granola has a fall feel to it, thanks to the pumpkin, hazelnut, and maple, it tastes divine all year long. Keep it stashed in your bag for emergencies or add it to your yogurt parfaits in the morning.

Makes 1¼ cups

¼ cup pepitas or roasted
   pumpkin squash seeds

¼ cup walnuts

¼ cup pecans

¼ cup hazelnuts

¼ cup pumpkin puree
   (NOT pumpkin pie filling)

2 tablespoons pure maple syrup

½ teaspoon pure vanilla extract

¼ teaspoon sea salt

Preheat the oven to 450°F.

Combine all of the ingredients in a large bowl and mix well. Spread over a baking sheet and bake for 15 minutes, or until the nuts are golden and fragrant. Allow the mixture to cool before storing in an airtight container for up to 2 weeks. Enjoy with a small piece of fruit, such as an apple or orange, if you want to add more color to your meal.

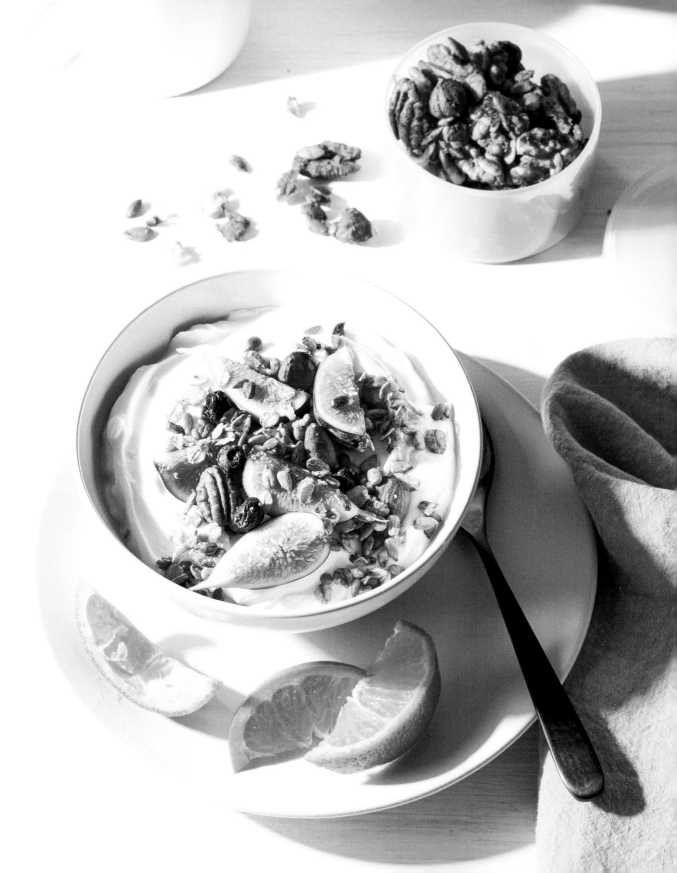

BERRY COCONUT CHIA PUDDING PARFAIT

Chia seeds are all the rage right now, and for good reason: These small but mighty seeds are packed with protein and when combined with liquid, they expand twenty-five times their weight to create a gel-like consistency that's perfect for giving your digestive system a clean sweep (which is amazing news for your gut). This creamy pudding also layers in fruit, yogurt, nuts, and hemp seeds for a snack that will give you a turbo boost of energy.

Serves 1

½ cup 2 percent plain Greek yogurt
 or nondairy yogurt

¼ cup unsweetened coconut milk
 or nut milk

1 tablespoon chia seeds

1 teaspoon pure maple syrup or
 raw honey

½ teaspoon pure vanilla extract

½ cup raspberries

¼ cup blackberries

¼ cup low-sugar, whole grain
 granola (such as Trail Mix
 Granola on page 216)

2 tablespoons pistachios

1 tablespoon hemp seeds

In a medium bowl, mix together the yogurt, milk, chia seeds, maple syrup or honey, and vanilla.

In a parfait glass or jar, layer the chia pudding with the fruit, granola, pistachios, and hemp seeds.

HOMEMADE HUMMUS

Chickpeas are a great source of plant protein, and this satisfying dip can be whipped up in minutes. If you're like our kids, you might find yourself eating it by the spoonful, but if you're adulting, then you'll love to pair it with raw veggies like cucumbers, bell peppers, carrots, cauliflower, jicama, sugar snap peas, and broccoli. Think of this as your hummus foundation and then doctor it up with any seasonings or flavors that bring you joy, such as some sautéed jalepeño peppers or a nice sprinkle of smoky paprika or cumin.

Makes 1½ cups

2 (15-ounce) cans chickpeas, drained and rinsed

3 to 4 garlic cloves, depending on how garlicky you like your hummus

¼ cup tahini

¼ cup fresh lemon juice

1½ tablespoons extra-virgin olive oil

Sea salt and freshly ground black pepper to taste

Unlimited colorful raw veggies, for serving

Combine all of the ingredients in a blender or food processor and blend until smooth. Store in an airtight container in the refrigerator for up to 1 week or freeze for up to 1 month.

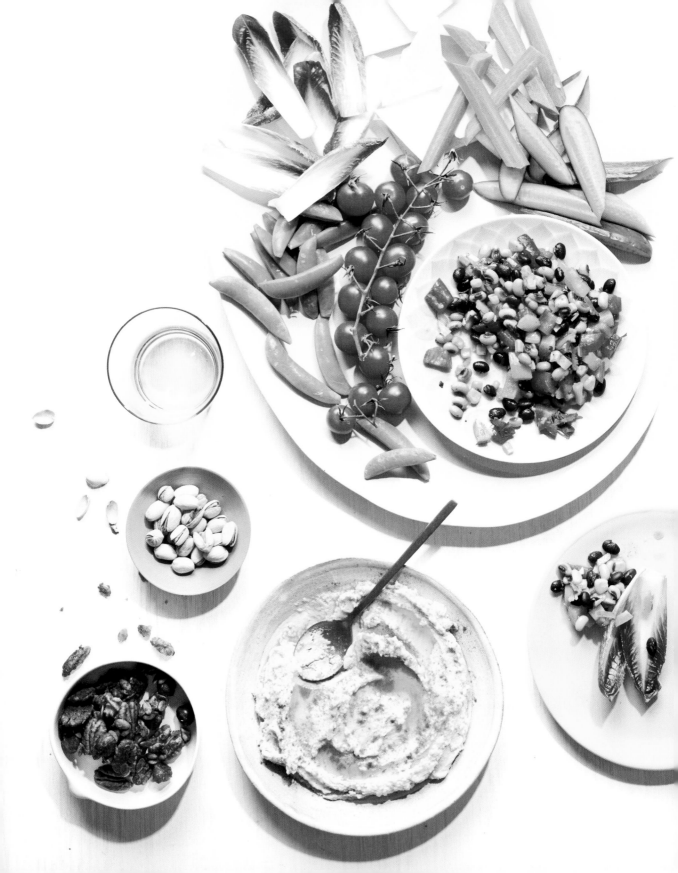

COWBOY CAVIAR

This easy-to-throw-together dip is super versatile—pack it up and take it to a party with a bag of chips, scoop it on top of your favorite salad, or serve with fresh veggies. Thanks to the protein and carbs from the legumes and the fat from the oil, this could also serve as a balanced meal on its own if all you had was a spoon!

Serves 6 to 8

1 (15-ounce) can black beans, rinsed and drained

1 (15-ounce) can black-eyed peas, rinsed and drained

1 cup frozen sweet corn, thawed

3 Roma tomatoes, diced

2 bell peppers (two different colors of your choice), cored, seeded, and diced

½ small red onion, diced

2 garlic cloves, minced

¼ cup roughly chopped fresh cilantro

¼ cup avocado oil

¼ cup apple cider vinegar

1 teaspoon ground cumin

¼ teaspoon cayenne

½ teaspoon sea salt

¼ teaspoon freshly ground black pepper

Place all of the ingredients in a large bowl and mix gently until combined. Store in the fridge for up to 3 days.

SUPER EGG SALAD

We are all about taking classic, comfort-food favorites and making them "super," or healthier, than the originals. In this case, we lightened things up by swapping out mayo for avocado and using more egg whites than yolks for an egg salad that's even more delicious than your standard variety. We love heaping this salad onto rice cakes, sprouted grain toast, or crackers.

Serves 2

4 hard-boiled eggs, chopped

2 hard-boiled egg whites, chopped

3 celery stalks, chopped

½ avocado, diced

1 Roma tomato, diced

2 green onions (white and green parts), chopped

1 tablespoon chopped fresh dill

1 teaspoon Dijon mustard

2 brown or wild rice cakes or 2 pieces sprouted grain toast

In a large bowl, combine all of the ingredients except the rice cakes and mix well. Serve over the rice cakes or toast.

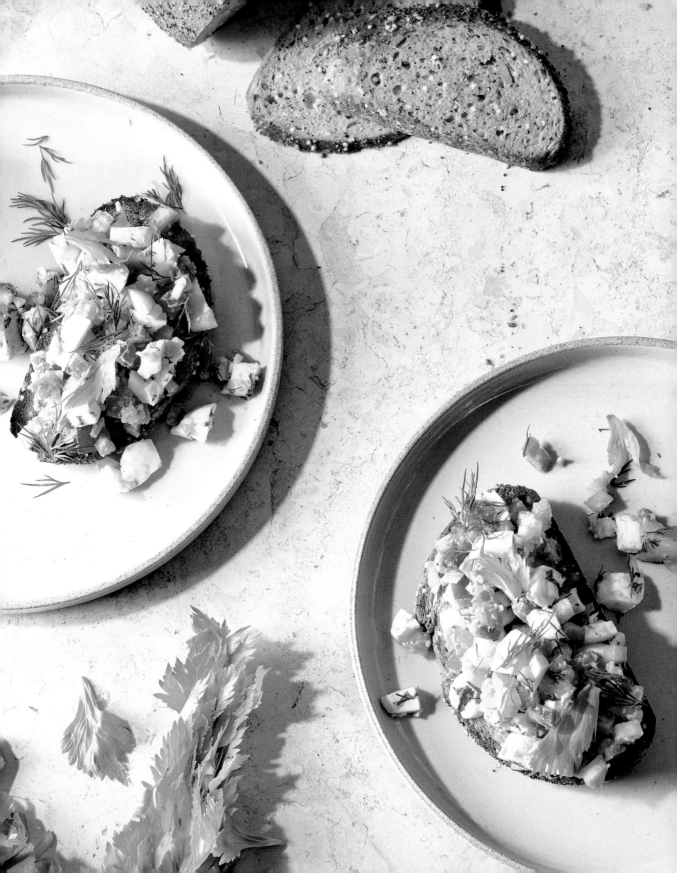

TRAIL MIX GRANOLA

This is somewhat of a spin-off from the Craving Crusher Granola (page 208), with the addition of a healthy grain to show you how much more delicious homemade granola is than store-bought (not to mention lower in sugar and way less expensive). Adding oats to the mix also means that this granola is a complete meal with a well-rounded combination of carbohydrates, fat, and protein—plus two colors from the pumpkin and dried berries.

Makes 8 to 10 (⅓-cup) servings

1 cup rolled oats

1 cup raw pecan halves or pieces

1 cup unsalted sunflower seeds

½ cup raw almonds

½ can pumpkin puree (NOT pumpkin pie filling)

¼ cup unsweetened dried berries

1 tablespoon raw honey

1 teaspoon pumpkin pie spice

Preheat the oven to 350°F. Line a large baking sheet with parchment paper or a silicone baking mat and set aside.

Combine all of the ingredients in a large bowl and mix well. Spread the mixture over the prepared baking sheet and bake for 20 minutes, or until the nuts are golden brown. Let the granola cool completely, then store in an airtight container at room temperature for up to 2 weeks.

APPLE NACHOS

This is a naturally sweet snack that our kids love to have after school—and so do we! If you don't have homemade granola on hand, feel free to use a lower-sugar store-bought version, like Purely Elizabeth.

Serves 1 to 2

1 apple, peeled, cored,
 and thinly sliced

2 tablespoons unsweetened almond
 butter, ideally slightly warmed

¼ cup granola, preferably
 homemade (page 216)

Arrange the apple slices on a plate, drizzle with the almond butter, and sprinkle with the granola.

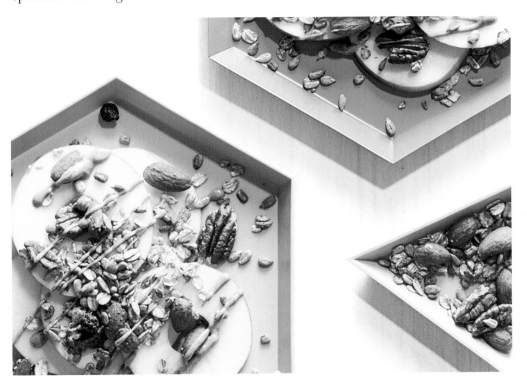

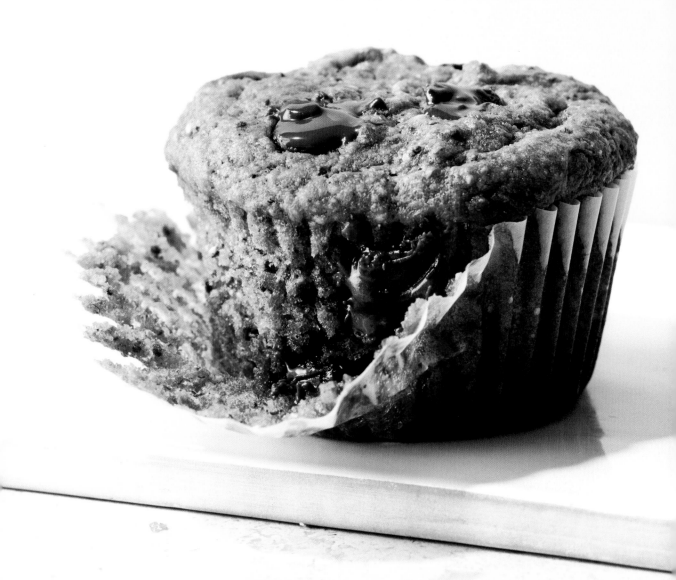

PEANUT BUTTER CHIA CHOCOLATE CHIP MUFFINS

Peanut butter and chocolate chips?! Don't worry, there's nothing naughty about these bite-sized snacks, which are perfect for eating on the run. Chia seeds and flax meal are not only fat and protein powerhouses that balance the sugar and carbs, but they're also loaded with omega-3s, which can be harder to get from plant-based foods. These fatty acids are what I like to call "brain food" and are also really beneficial for your digestive system.

Makes 12 to 16 muffins

2 frozen bananas, thawed and
   mashed (with liquid)

1 cup unsweetened peanut butter

3 large eggs, beaten

¼ cup unsweetened almond milk

1 teaspoon pure vanilla extract

⅓ cup coconut flour

¼ cup coconut sugar

2 tablespoons chia seeds

1 tablespoon flax meal

1 teaspoon ground cinnamon

1 teaspoon baking soda

⅓ cup dark chocolate chips

Preheat the oven to 350°F. Line 12 to 16 wells of a muffin tin with paper cups and set aside.

In a large bowl, combine the bananas, peanut butter, eggs, almond milk, and vanilla. Mix well.

In a second large bowl, combine the flour, sugar, chia seeds, flax meal, cinnamon, and baking soda. Mix well.

Gradually add the dry ingredients to the wet and mix until well combined. Fold in the chocolate chips. Divide the batter among the muffin cups, filling them three-quarters full. Bake for 20 to 25 minutes, until a toothpick or knife inserted in the center comes out clean. Cool completely and store in the fridge for up to 5 days.

Lunch

CALIFORNIA CHICKEN BOWL

As you know by now, we both are creatures of habit and happily eat the same things over and over, and this salad is frequently in rotation at both of our houses. It's hearty and filling, thanks to marinated chicken and brown rice, plus tons of cooked veggies and lots of colors. If you don't eat animal protein, feel free to sub in lentils or beans.

Serves 4

For the grilled chicken:

¼ cup extra-virgin olive oil

¼ cup chopped fresh parsley or 1 tablespoon dried

¼ cup chopped fresh basil or 1 tablespoon dried

4 garlic cloves, minced

½ teaspoon onion powder

½ teaspoon smoked paprika

½ teaspoon freshly ground black pepper, plus more to taste

¼ teaspoon cayenne pepper

1 pound boneless skinless chicken breast or tenders, cubed if using skewers

To assemble:

1½ cups uncooked brown rice

2 red bell peppers, cored, seeded, and quartered

1 medium zucchini, sliced into ¼-inch rounds

1 tablespoon extra-virgin olive oil

Sea salt and freshly ground black pepper

2 avocados, mashed well

Juice of 1 lemon

½ cup chopped fresh parsley

1 garlic clove, minced

1 pint grape tomatoes, halved, for serving

Walnut pieces, for serving

(cont.)

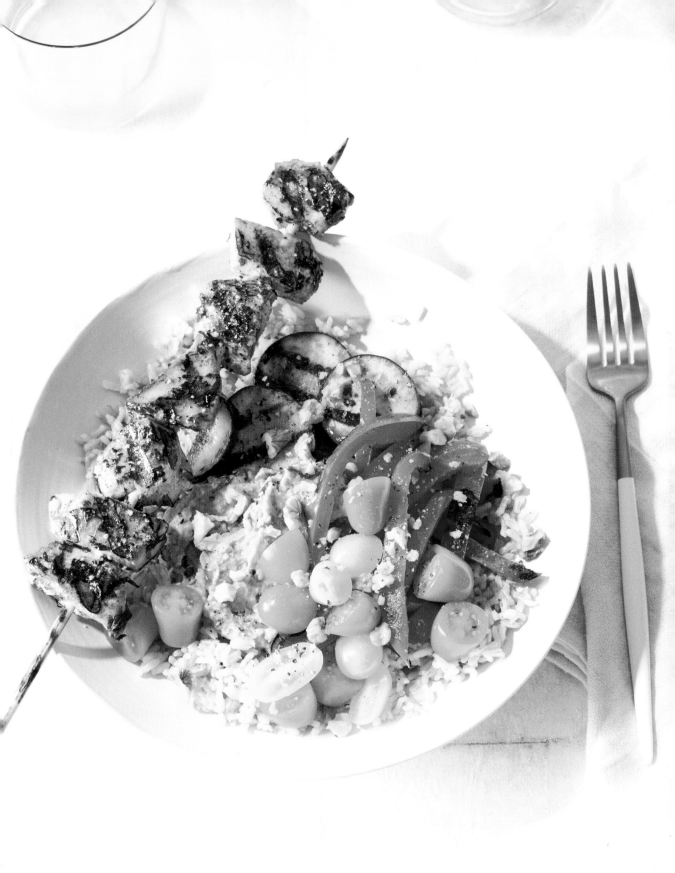

If using bamboo sewers, let them soak in water for at least 30 minutes before grilling the chicken. (This will prevent them from charring.)

TO MARINATE THE CHICKEN: In a large bowl, combine the olive oil, parsley, basil, garlic, onion powder, paprika, black pepper, and cayenne. Add the chicken and toss well. Cover the bowl with plastic wrap and refrigerate while you prepare the rest of the meal.

Fill a medium pot with 3 cups of filtered water and bring to a boil. Reduce the heat to medium and add the rice. Stir to combine, cover the pot with a lid, and reduce the heat to the lowest setting possible. Cook for 10 minutes, then turn off the heat. Let the rice sit, covered, for 20 minutes. (Don't take any peeks inside!) Remove the lid and fluff the rice with a fork. Cover to keep warm and set aside.

Preheat a grill, grill pan, or large sauté pan to medium-high heat. Place the red peppers and zucchini in a gallon-sized zip-top bag. Add 1 tablespoon of the olive oil plus a pinch of salt and pepper. Seal the bag and shake well so the veggies are well coated. Set aside.

Divide the chicken among the skewers and lay them on the grill or pan. If not using skewers, lay the whole breasts on the grill. Cook for 3 to 4 minutes per side, carefully flipping 2 or 3 times, until the chicken is cooked through and has light char marks.

While the chicken is cooking, add the zucchini and red peppers to the grill or pan. Cook for 4 to 5 minutes on each side, until the veggies are tender.

Remove everything from the grill or pan and let cool for 5 minutes. Meanwhile, in a large bowl, combine the mashed avocados with the lemon juice, parsley, and garlic. Season with salt and pepper.

Slice the peppers into thin strips, and if you left the chicken breasts whole, cut them into cubes. Assemble the bowls by dividing the rice among 4 bowls. Top the rice with equal amounts of chicken, grilled veggies, and a large dollop of the avocado mixture. Serve warm with tomatoes and walnuts.

HUMMUS POWER BOWL

We're all used to eating hummus as a dip, but this nutrient-packed lunch is the perfect way to incorporate a favorite food in a whole new way—it's basically like transforming veggies and dip into a salad bowl. We like to use our Homemade Hummus (page 211) in this lunch, but if you are buying your hummus, be sure to read the label carefully. You want to choose a brand made with olive, sunflower seed, or sesame oil, not canola oil. You also want to make sure there aren't any ingredients you don't recognize or can't pronounce!

Serves 2

½ cup cauliflower rice

½ cup shredded carrots

1 cup chopped cucumber

½ cup hummus

4 tablespoons pepitas

Cayenne pepper, for serving (optional)

Chopped fresh parsley, for serving (optional)

Make a bed of the cauliflower rice, carrots, and cucumber in the bottom of two bowls. Top each with half of the hummus and the pepitas. Sprinkle with a pinch of cayenne pepper and parsley, if desired.

FERMENTED CUCUMBER SALAD

This salad is not only delicious, but it also delivers lots of fermented goodness to your gut. Fermented foods—or foods whose carbohydrates have been broken down by beneficial bacteria— supply your microbiome with good-for-you flora and enzymes, strengthening your digestive system and making your food and its nutrients more readily absorbed. This salad makes a great lunch (feel free to top with a protein of your choice) or a side dish for dinner.

Serves 4

1 medium cucumber, sliced or chopped

½ cup sauerkraut or kimchi

1 medium tomato, diced

¼ cup diced red onion

½ cup corn kernels

1 tablespoon extra-virgin olive oil

Sea salt and black pepper, to taste

2 tablespoons nutritional yeast

1 teaspoon hemp seeds

In a large bowl, toss together all of the salad ingredients. Top with the protein of your choice, if desired, and enjoy.

STRAWBERRY TOSSED SALAD

This is a not-to-be-missed salad during fresh strawberry season, between late spring and early summer. You hardly need to dress the berries because they're so sweet and juicy, and as far as macros go, you're all set, even if you don't add the chicken. Plus, it's packed with fiber, which will help keep you feeling satisfied between meals. Feel free to get creative on greens—spinach or arugula would also be delicious here!

Serves 1

For the dressing:

Juice of 1 lemon

1 tablespoon extra-virgin olive oil

1 teaspoon honey (preferably raw
or Manuka)

Sea salt and freshly ground black
pepper to taste

For the salad:

1 cup romaine lettuce

1 cup spring mix

½ cup diced cucumber

½ cup sliced strawberries

¼ cup shredded carrots

¼ cup corn kernels

¼ cup slivered almonds
(toasted, if desired)

4 ounces cooked chicken
breast (optional)

TO MAKE THE DRESSING: In a small bowl, whisk together the lemon juice, oil, honey, salt, and pepper.

In a large bowl, toss together all of the salad ingredients. Drizzle with the dressing and enjoy.

CUCUMBER RIBBON SALAD

After you finish the Reset and your skin is radiant with renewed health, people are going to be asking you all the time what your secret is. We suggest sharing this simple yet impressive-looking dish made with hydrating cucumber. Besides spiralizing or thinly shaving the cucumber, there's nothing more to it than tossing the ingredients together, but your friends will be wowed!

Serves 4

¼ cup apple cider vinegar

2 tablespoons extra-virgin olive oil

1 teaspoon raw honey or pure maple syrup

1 teaspoon chopped fresh dill

2 cups radishes, thinly sliced

1 English cucumber, spiralized using the ribbon blade (or peeled into "noodles" with a flat peeler)

1 cup sliced bell pepper (colors of your choice)

¼ cup finely sliced green onion (white and green parts)

Sea salt and freshly ground black pepper, to taste

In a large bowl, whisk together the vinegar, oil, honey or maple syrup, and dill. Add the veggies and toss gently to coat. Season with salt and pepper to taste.

GREEK POTATO SALAD

People are always surprised to learn that they can eat potatoes on Cara's program. First of all, the Wellness Remodel doesn't exclude any foods unless they don't make you feel good. Second, potatoes are a great source of the starches and carbohydrates that your body needs to thrive. And they, like all other plants, have their own unique benefits like vitamins C and B_6, potassium, and magnesium, plus lots of fiber.

This recipe is a remodeled version of the classic summer favorite. We added fresh herbs and fresh greens, as well as a handful of Kalamata olives (or chopped avocado, if you prefer), which are a great source of healthy fat and will keep the carbohydrate-rich potatoes from spiking your blood sugar.

Serves 4

12 small red potatoes, halved

2 cups cherry tomatoes, halved

1 cup finely chopped red onion

¼ cup nutritional yeast

15 pitted Kalamata olives or 1 large avocado, chopped

1 cup spinach, chopped

¼ cup minced fresh dill

¼ cup minced fresh parsley

¼ cup fresh lemon juice

2 tablespoons extra-virgin olive oil

Sea salt and freshly ground black pepper

2 tablespoons toasted pine nuts, for garnish

Place the potatoes in a large pot and add enough cold water just to cover. Bring to a boil, reduce to a simmer, and cook until fork-tender, about 15 minutes. Strain and let the potatoes cool slightly.

While potatoes are cooking, combine the tomatoes, red onion, nutritional yeast, and olives or avocado in a large bowl. Add the cooked potatoes and fold in the spinach, dill, parsley, lemon juice, and oil. Toss well, season with salt and pepper, and sprinkle with the pine nuts before serving.

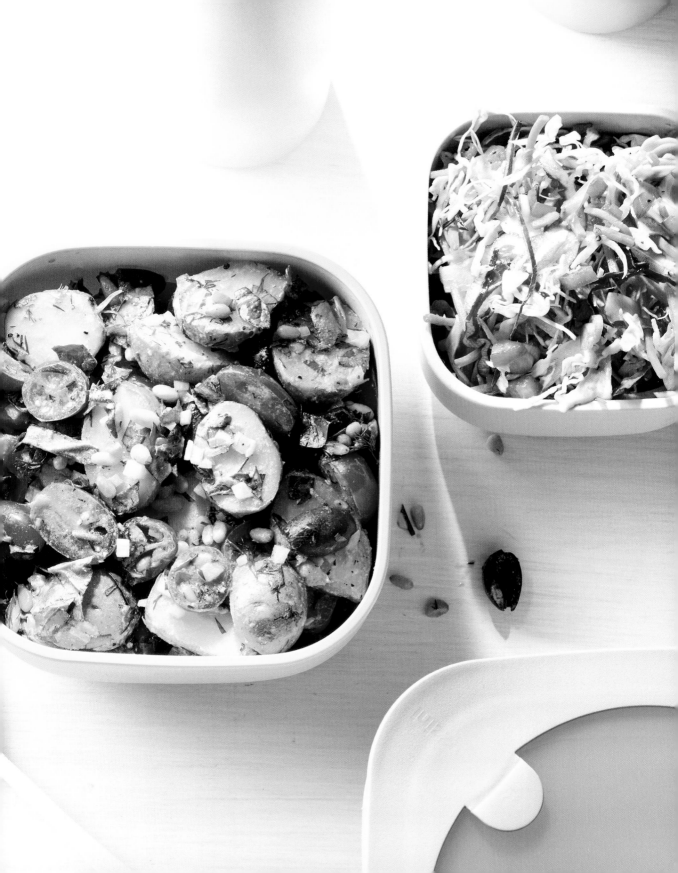

CRUNCHY COLESLAW

This is one of our favorite salads to bring to summer barbecues—it's always a hit. But it's easy enough to make that you don't need to wait for a special occasion . . . you can enjoy it any day of the week. The biggest bonus is that you're getting all five colors at once, especially if you can find a shredded cabbage or coleslaw mix that has both green and red cabbage (or you shred them yourself).

Serves 6

2 (12-ounce) bags shredded cabbage or coleslaw mix

1 (12-ounce) bag shredded carrots

8 green onions, sliced (white and greens parts)

1 large green bell pepper, cored, seeded, and diced

½ cup slivered almonds (toasted for deeper flavor)

¼ cup balsamic vinegar

¼ cup extra-virgin olive oil

Kosher salt and freshly ground black pepper

In a large bowl, combine the cabbage, carrots, green onions, bell pepper, and almonds. Give everything a toss and drizzle with the vinegar and olive oil to coat everything well. Season to taste with salt and pepper.

TACO SALAD

Getting your taco fix doesn't mean you need to eat a greasy meal that leaves you feeling heavy and bloated. This single-serving salad scratches the itch and fills you up with a rainbow of nutri-ents It's also a great way to use up any leftover mango salsa from a dinner of Coconut Shrimp Tacos (page 245) the next day!

Serves 1

4 ounces cooked chicken or ½ cup cooked pinto beans

2 cups chopped romaine lettuce

¼ cup sweet corn kernels

5 to 6 grape or cherry tomatoes

¼ cup mango salsa (page 245) or store-bought salsa

¼ avocado, chopped

Lime wedge, for serving

Layer the ingredients in a bowl, top with a squeeze of lime, and dig in.

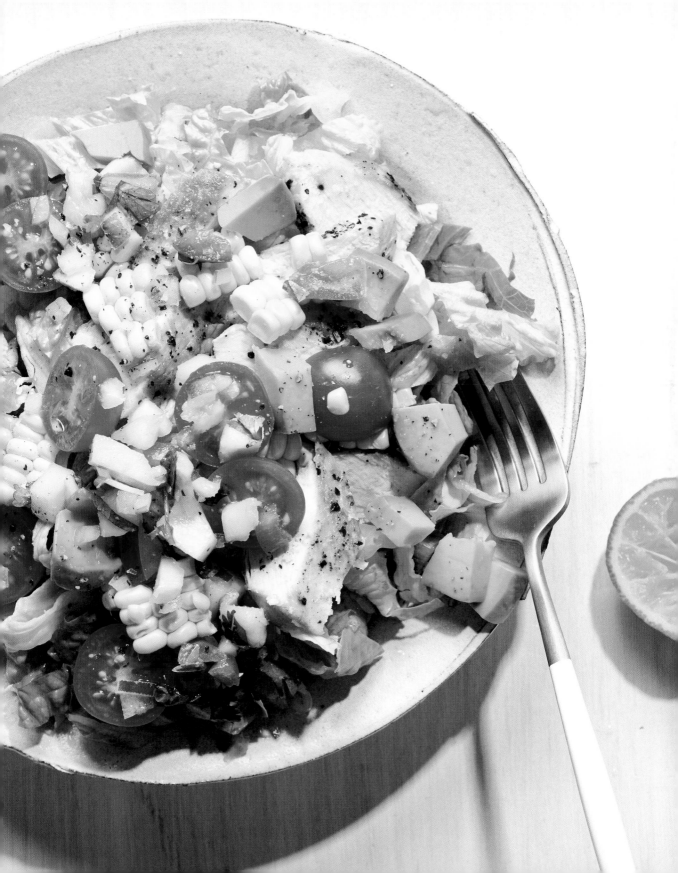

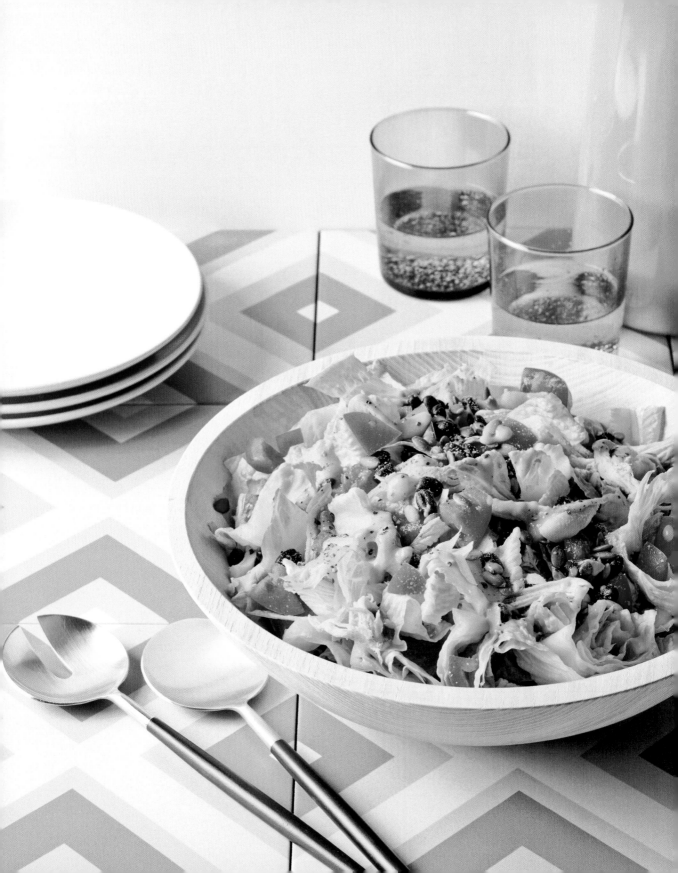

MEXICAN CAESAR SALAD

This twist on the classic Caesar borrows bright flavors from Mexican cooking. The perfectly creamy avocado-lime dressing is to die for, and gets topped with a sprinkle of nutritional yeast, which has a salty, cheese-like flavor and is packed with vitamins and minerals that help strengthen your immune system. If you want to make this vegetarian, just leave off the chicken and double the amount of black beans.

Serves 1

For the avocado-lime dressing:
½ avocado
Juice of 1 lime, plus more if needed
1 tablespoon nutritional yeast
Sea salt and freshly ground black
   pepper

For the salad:
2 cups chopped romaine lettuce
4 ounces shredded chicken breast
½ cup chopped fresh cilantro
¼ cup cooked black beans
1 small Roma tomato, chopped
2 tablespoons pepitas (toast for
   more flavor)
1 to 2 tablespoons
   nutritional yeast

In a blender, combine the avocado, lime juice, and nutritional yeast and blend until smooth. Season with salt and pepper. If you need to thin the dressing, add a touch more lime juice or water.

In a large bowl, toss together the salad ingredients and drizzle with the dressing.

LOADED DELI SANDWICH

We're not here to act like we never eat a sammy! We just do it a little differently. Healthy fat, protein, and plenty of veggies are piled onto sprouted grain bread with a little hit of something salty-sweet, like sauerkraut, pickles, or even kimchi if you like some heat. Feel free to customize with any lean protein you have on hand—sliced chicken breast or even a veggie burger patty would work well, too.

Serves 1

2 slices Ezekiel or other sprouted
   wheat bread, or gluten-free bread

1 tablespoon yellow mustard

¼ avocado, sliced or mashed

4 ounces turkey breast

¼ cup sprouts

2 romaine lettuce leaves

¼ cup sauerkraut or pickles
   of choice

1 slice tomato

1 tablespoon sunflower seeds

Spread the mustard over one slice of bread and the avocado over the other. Layer one slice with the turkey, sprouts, lettuce, sauerkraut or pickles, tomato, and sunflower seeds, then close that baby up and enjoy!

KITCHEN SINK SALAD

This is one of those "everybody in the pool" kinda deals—it's a great way to use up any produce left in the crisper at the end of the week and it's always satisfying. Plus you won't have to worry about getting in your five colors! Done and done. To keep things easy, we used lemon juice plus salt and pepper as a light dressing, but if you have any extra lemon-tahini dressing (see page 237) on hand, it also works well here.

Serves 1

2 cups mixed greens

3 to 4 ounces cooked chicken breast
  or ½ cup cooked beans

½ cup chopped or shredded
  cabbage

¼ cup shredded carrot

¼ avocado, diced

¼ cup corn kernels

¼ cup diced strawberries

Unlimited chopped cucumber,
  bell pepper, and tomato

2 tablespoons chopped walnuts

Fresh lemon juice

Sea salt and freshly ground
  black pepper

In a large bowl, combine the salad ingredients. Sprinkle with the lemon juice and a pinch of salt and pepper and toss to combine.

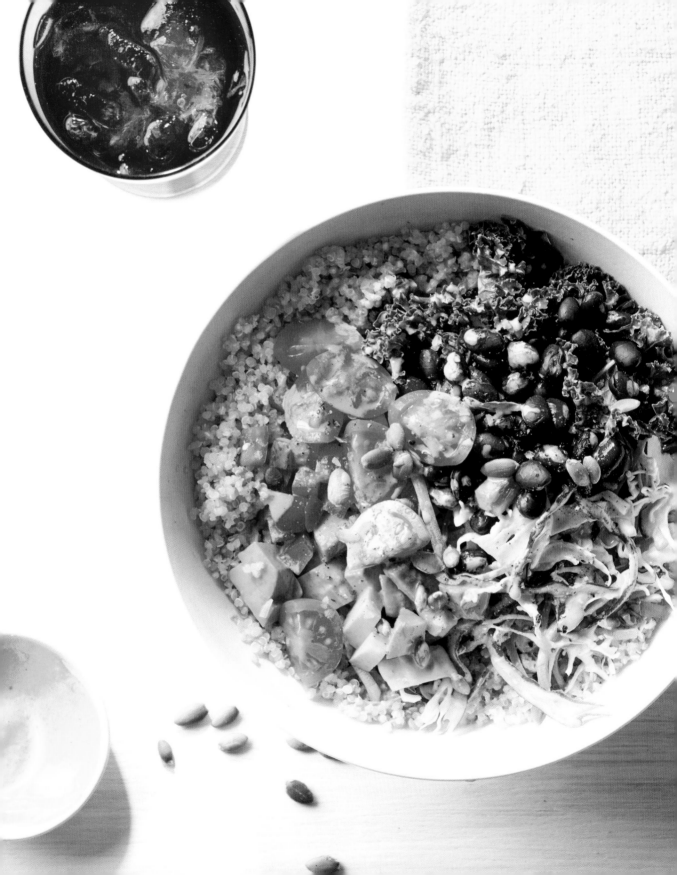

QUINOA BOWL

When it comes to grains, many nutritionists recommend enjoying ½ to ¾ cup at a meal. But when it comes to quinoa, which is actually a seed, that serving increases to 1 cup, if you like. A cup of quinoa packs close to 9 grams of protein—about as much as a cup of yogurt. The lemon-tahini dressing we drizzle on this bowl is super delicious, but if you're pressed for time, you can skip it—a good, creamy avocado will also do the trick!

Serves 1

1 cup cooked quinoa

Handful of spinach or kale leaves

Handful of sliced cabbage or slaw mix (bonus points for carrots or broccoli in there!)

¼ avocado, diced

¼ cup diced bell pepper (color of your choice)

5 cherry or grape tomatoes

¼ cup cooked black beans, lightly seasoned with salt

Handful of sprouts (optional)

2 tablespoons pepitas or sunflower seeds (toasted for best flavor)

For the lemon-tahini dressing (optional):

½ tablespoon tahini

1 tablespoon fresh lemon juice

¼ teaspoon garlic powder

¼ to ½ teaspoon hot sauce (optional)

Dash of ground turmeric

Sea salt and freshly ground black pepper to taste

Layer the ingredients in a large bowl and enjoy! If making the dressing, combine the ingredients in a medium bowl and whisk with 1 tablespoon of water. Toss with the salad.

Dinner

CHICKEN ZUCCHINI BURGERS

The all-American burger dinner is one of our favorites, but that doesn't mean it has to include beef, which is high in saturated fat and often contains added hormones, thanks to unhealthy farming practices. We'll enjoy a nice serving of grass-fed beef every once in a while, but when it comes to everyday dinners, chicken makes a great alternative for a thick, juicy burger. Add some shredded veggies (the kids'll never know they're there!) and a tangy Greek yogurt sauce, and you've got a dinner the whole family will get excited about!

Serves 4

For the Greek yogurt sauce:
1 cup 2 percent plain Greek yogurt
2 teaspoons lemon zest
2 tablespoons fresh lemon juice
2 garlic cloves, minced
1 tablespoon extra-virgin olive oil
½ teaspoon sea salt

For the burgers:
1 pound ground chicken or turkey breast

1 medium zucchini, shredded, excess water squeezed out with a clean kitchen towel or cheesecloth
½ cup corn kernels
½ medium red bell pepper, cored, seeded, and finely chopped
3 green onions (white and green parts), thinly sliced
1 large egg, lightly beaten
½ cup whole wheat panko bread crumbs or almond flour
2 tablespoons chopped fresh cilantro

(cont.)

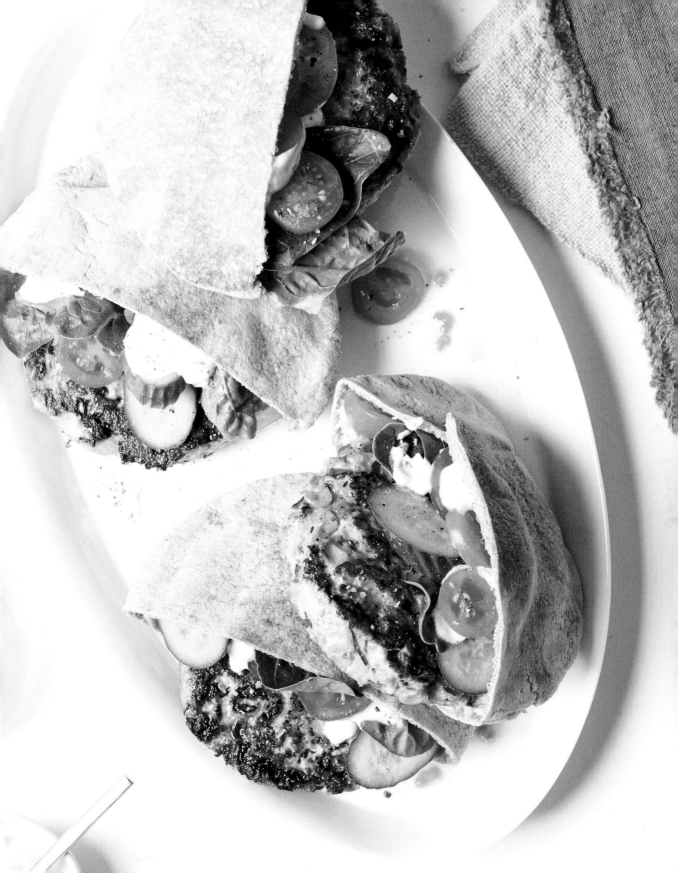

3 garlic cloves, finely chopped

1 teaspoon ground cumin

1 teaspoon kosher salt

½ teaspoon freshly ground black pepper

2 tablespoons avocado oil

For serving:

2 whole grain pitas, halved into pockets

¼ cup hummus, homemade (page 211) or store-bought

Romaine lettuce or spinach

Chopped cucumber

Sliced tomatoes

Make the Greek yogurt sauce by mixing together all of the ingredients in a small bowl. Place in the fridge until ready to serve.

Preheat the oven to 425°F.

In a large bowl, combine all of the burger ingredients except the oil. Use your hands to mix well and form 4 patties.

Heat the oil in a large ovenproof skillet over medium heat, swirling to coat the bottom of the pan. Add the patties and sear for about 2 minutes on each side until golden brown. Carefully transfer the pan to the oven and bake for 7 to 10 minutes, until cooked through.

While the burgers are baking, smear about a tablespoon of hummus inside each pita pocket. Stuff with the veggies and top with the cooked burgers. Either drizzle the Greek yogurt sauce inside or serve it as a dip.

PINEAPPLE STIR-FRY

This dish definitely falls in the don't-knock-it-'til-you've-tried-it category. I know adding pineapple to a savory dish can seems strange—though I'm no stranger than Hawaiian pizza—but when the fruit heats through, its sweetness gets much more mellow and deepens the savory flavors of the vegetables. All those complex notes plus lots of fresh herbs (you can choose your favorite) makes for a restaurant-caliber dish.

Serves 4

1 tablespoon coconut oil

¼ teaspoon crushed red pepper flakes

1 medium pineapple, cored and diced

1 head of broccoli, chopped into small florets

1 medium red bell pepper, cored, seeded, and sliced

1 small onion, sliced

Sea salt and freshly ground black pepper, to taste

2 cups cooked chicken or turkey breast, diced into 1-inch pieces, or 1 pound cooked medium wild shrimp

¼ cup fresh leafy herbs of your choice (parsley, cilantro, basil)

2 tablespoons toasted sesame seeds, for garnish (optional)

½ cup cooked wild rice or quinoa, for serving (optional)

In a large skillet over medium-high heat, melt the coconut oil. Add the crushed red pepper flakes and sauté for about 1 minute before adding the pineapple, broccoli, bell pepper, and onion. Season with salt and pepper and cook until the veggies are tender and most of the pineapple juice has cooked off, 5 to 6 minutes. Stir in the chicken or turkey or shrimp and the herbs and cook until heated through, about 2 minutes. Taste and adjust the seasoning with more salt and pepper, if desired. Top with toasted sesame seeds, if desired, and serve with rice or quinoa.

SALMON & VEGGIES

We all need a little more basic in our lives—things that are unfussy and dependably deliver without being overcomplicated. This dish is just that. It's a great weeknight meal because it comes together so easily (wrapping the salmon in parchment with basil and lemon guarantees that the fish will be perfectly cooked and flavorful every time) and kids love it, too.

Serves 4

4 (4-ounce) salmon fillets

Sea salt and freshly ground black pepper to taste

¼ cup chopped fresh basil

2 tablespoons avocado oil

2 lemons, thinly sliced

3 cups cauliflower florets, chopped

¼ cup diced red onion

1¼ cup pistachios

3 tablespoons nutritional yeast

Preheat the oven to 350°F. Cut 4 15-inch by 15-inch square pieces of parchment and set aside.

Season the salmon with salt and pepper. Use a knife to slice 2½-inch slices into the flesh of each piece of salmon, taking care not to cut all the way through the fish. Tuck the basil into each of the slits. Place one piece of salmon on each of the parchment squares. Drizzle each piece of salmon with 1 teaspoon of the avocado oil and place the lemon slices on top.

Gather up the sides of the parchment over the fish to form a pouch with no openings. Place the packets on a baking sheet and cook for 20 minutes.

While the salmon cooks, heat a skillet over medium heat. Add the remaining 2 teaspoons of the avocado oil and sauté the cauliflower until tender, about 20 minutes. Add the onion and season with salt and pepper. Continue cooking until the onions begin to brown, about 10 minutes. Remove the pan from the heat and toss with the pistachios and nutritional yeast.

QUICK CANNELLINI & SPINACH PASTA

The best thing about this meal is how quickly it can be put together and yet how polished it is when it's done. Not to mention the fact that the beans pack close to 10 grams of fiber per serving and about 7 grams of protein—awesome news for our plant-based friends.

Serves 4

8 ounces whole grain penne or rotini pasta

1 tablespoon avocado oil

8 ounces baby spinach

3 garlic cloves, chopped

1 to 2 teaspoons red pepper flakes (depending on how much heat you like)

1 (28-ounce) can crushed tomatoes

Sea salt and freshly ground black pepper to taste

1 (15-ounce) can of cannellini beans, rinsed and drained

1 (6.5-ounce) jar of marinated artichokes, drained and roughly chopped

1 (2.25-ounce) can of sliced black olives, rinsed and drained

Freshly grated Parmesan cheese or nutritional yeast, for serving (optional)

In a medium pot, bring 5 cups of water to a boil over medium-high heat. Add the pasta and cook for 2 minutes less than the package instructions advise (it will continue to cook once it's added to the sauce). Drain and set aside.

In a large pan over medium heat, add the avocado oil and sauté the spinach until just wilted, about 2 minutes. Transfer the spinach to a bowl and add the garlic and red pepper flakes to the pan. Cook until fragrant, about 1 minute, then add the tomatoes. Season with salt and pepper, reduce the heat to medium, and simmer for 15 to 20 minutes, until the flavors have come together and the sauce has thickened slightly.

Add the pasta to the pan, along with the sautéed spinach, beans, artichokes, and olives. Cook for another 1 to 2 minutes until everything is warmed through and the pasta is al dente. Serve sprinkled with the Parmesan or nutritional yeast, if desired.

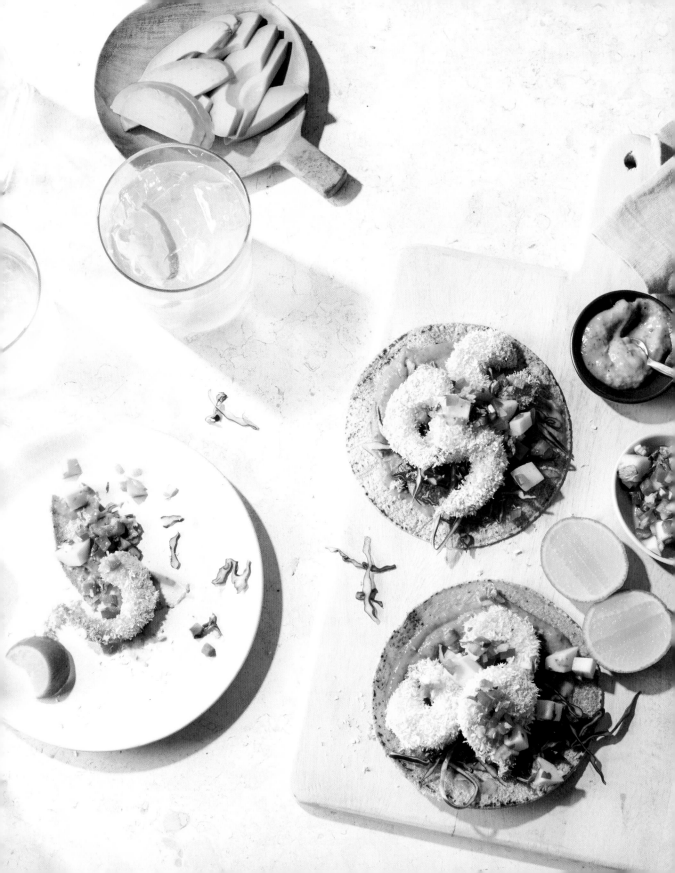

COCONUT SHRIMP TACOS WITH MANGO SALSA AND AVOCADO CILANTRO SAUCE

This dish is so easy to make and yet looks and tastes impressive enough to serve for a dinner party. The salsa is really what makes the dish sing—you might want to double the recipe so you have leftovers for dipping with chips or using in our Taco Salad (page 230).

Serves 4

For the shrimp:

Coconut or avocado oil cooking spray

1 cup unsweetened shredded coconut

½ teaspoon paprika

Sea salt and freshly ground black pepper

1 egg

1 pound medium wild shrimp, peeled, deveined, and tails removed

For the salsa:

1 cup diced mango or pineapple

½ cup diced red bell pepper

¼ cup diced red onion

Zest and juice of 1 medium lime

2 tablespoons chopped fresh cilantro or mint

For the sauce:

1 cup loosely packed fresh cilantro

1 medium avocado

Juice of 1 medium lime

1 garlic clove

½ teaspoon ground cumin

Pinch of cayenne

Sea salt and freshly ground black pepper

For serving:

Small (gluten-free) corn tortillas or lettuce cups, finely shredded purple cabbage, avocado slices

Preheat the oven to 400°F. Place a wire rack on top of a large baking sheet, coat with cooking spray, and set aside.

(cont.)

In a medium bowl, mix together the coconut and paprika and season with salt and pepper. In a small bowl, whisk the egg with 1 tablespoon water.

Make an assembly line with the shrimp, egg wash, coconut mixture, and prepared baking sheet. Dip the shrimp in the egg wash, then dredge in the coconut, lightly shaking off any excess, then place the coated shrimp on the baking rack. Repeat with the remaining shrimp, spacing them out evenly on the baking rack so they will get crispy instead of steaming.

Bake for 12 to 14 minutes, until the shrimp are cooked through and the coconut has started to brown.

While the shrimp are cooking, make the salsa and sauce. In a medium bowl, toss together the salsa ingredients and set aside.

In a food processor or high-powered blender, add the sauce ingredients and ⅓ cup water. Pulse until smooth, adjusting the seasonings to your taste. If desired, spoon the sauce into a small zip-top bag and cut the tip off of one of the bottom corners (like you would to make a piping bag for icing), just enough to make a small hole. This will make it easier to drizzle your sauce more evenly, but you could also just use a spoon.

To assemble the tacos, place 3 to 4 shrimp on a tortilla or lettuce cup, top with shredded cabbage, a spoonful of salsa, and an avocado slice. Pipe or drizzle the sauce over the top.

SUMMER LOVIN' QUINOA BOWLS

You might be inclined to think that coconut, raisins, and mango have no place in a savory salad, but let us be the first to tell you just how deliciously satisfying the sweet-savory combo is here. It keeps this protein-packed meal feeling nice and light, while providing a hefty dose of macronutrients.

Serves 4

¼ cup balsamic vinegar

Zest and juice of 1 lime

2 cups cooked quinoa

1 cup cooked black beans

2 to 3 ounces cooked chicken (optional)

1 mango, peeled and diced

1 bell pepper (color of your choice), cored, seeded, and diced

⅓ cup chopped green onion (white and green parts)

¼ cup raisins

3 tablespoons unsweetened coconut flakes

Sea salt and freshly ground black pepper

Fresh cilantro, for garnish

In a small bowl, whisk together the balsamic vinegar, lime zest, and lime juice.

In a large bowl, combine the quinoa, black beans, chicken (if using), mango, bell pepper, green onion, raisins, and coconut flakes. Pour over the balsamic mixture and gently toss to combine. Season with salt and pepper and garnish with cilantro.

LOADED VEGGIE WHITE CHILI

This (shockingly) quick and easy meal—which you could also make in a slow cooker—is perfect for cooler days. The chili gets amazing depth of flavor from all the different vegetables and spices (without being spicy, per se), and always keeps you wanting more because it's so hearty that it's almost impossible to eat too much of it. We like to serve it with a variety of toppings—diced avocado, crushed corn tortilla chips, chopped fresh cilantro, lime wedges, pickled jalapeño slices—and let every member of the family pick their favorites or "decorate" their bowls.

Serves 8

1½ pounds chicken tenderloins (optional)

2 (15-ounce) cans cannellini beans, rinsed and drained

1 (15-ounce) can pinto beans, rinsed and drained

2 (4-ounce) cans diced green chilies

1 medium white onion, chopped

1 zucchini, chopped (optional)

1 green bell pepper, cored, seeded, and chopped

1 poblano pepper, cored, seeded, and chopped (optional)

2 jalapeños, minced (seeds removed for less spiciness, if desired)

3 garlic cloves, chopped

1 tablespoon chopped fresh oregano

1 tablespoon ground cumin

1 tablespoon chili powder

4 cups low-sodium chicken bone broth (if you can't find bone broth, chicken broth is fine)

Pinch of sea salt and freshly ground black pepper

Optional toppings: diced avocado, crushed corn tortilla chips, chopped fresh cilantro, lime wedges, pickled jalapeño slices

(cont.)

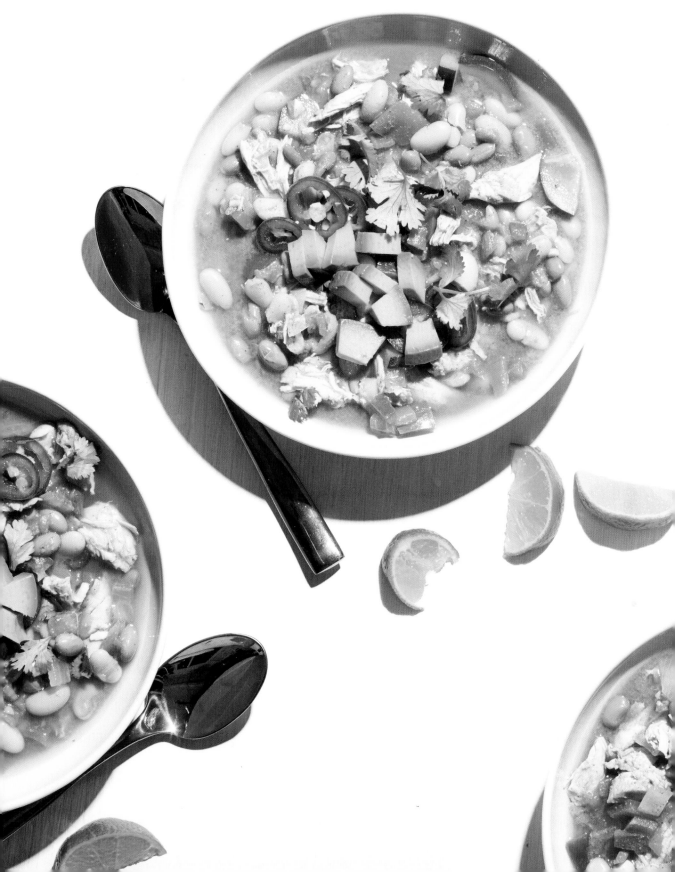

On the stovetop:

Combine all of the ingredients (except the toppings) in a large pot over medium-high heat. Bring the mixture to a boil and reduce to a simmer. Let the chili cook, uncovered, stirring occasionally, for 30 minutes if you haven't included the chicken, 45 minutes if you have.

In a slow cooker:

Combine all of the ingredients (except the toppings) in a slow cooker and cook on low for 4 to 5 hours, stirring occasionally.

If you've added the chicken, remove the pieces before serving and shred them with two forks. Return the shredded chicken to the chili and stir to combine. You may want to gently mash the beans with a potato masher for a thicker texture. Taste and adjust the seasoning with more salt and pepper if desired. Serve with your favorite toppings.

CHICKEN TORTILLA SOUP

This soup is deliciously fortifying, easy to make, and, best of all, freezes well so you can always have a batch on hand. To save time, you can use already cooked chicken breast and season it with the taco seasoning mix. Taco seasoning is super simple to make at home, but if you pick some up at the store, just make sure you choose a low-sodium version with no preservatives or MSG.

Serves 8 to 10

For the taco seasoning mix:

3 tablespoons ground cumin

1 tablespoon garlic powder

1 tablespoon chili powder

¼ to 1 teaspoon cayenne pepper (depending on how spicy you like it)

1 teaspoon sea salt

¼ teaspoon ground black pepper

For the soup:

Olive oil cooking spray (optional)

2 boneless skinless chicken breasts, halved

3 tablespoons taco seasoning mix, homemade (see above) or store-bought

5 small corn tortillas, sliced into thin strips

1 tablespoon avocado oil

3 bell peppers (choose 3 different colors), cored, seeded, and chopped

1 Vidalia onion, diced

4 garlic cloves, minced

1 (28-ounce) can no-salt-added fire-roasted diced tomatoes

3 tablespoons no-salt-added tomato paste

1 (15-ounce) can black beans, drained and rinsed

1 cup frozen sweet corn kernels, thawed

1 cup hominy (rinsed and drained, if from a can)

2 (4-ounce) cans diced green chilies

8 cups low-sodium chicken broth

Optional toppings: diced avocado, fresh cilantro, diced red onion, shredded Monterey Jack cheese, a squeeze of lime juice

(cont.)

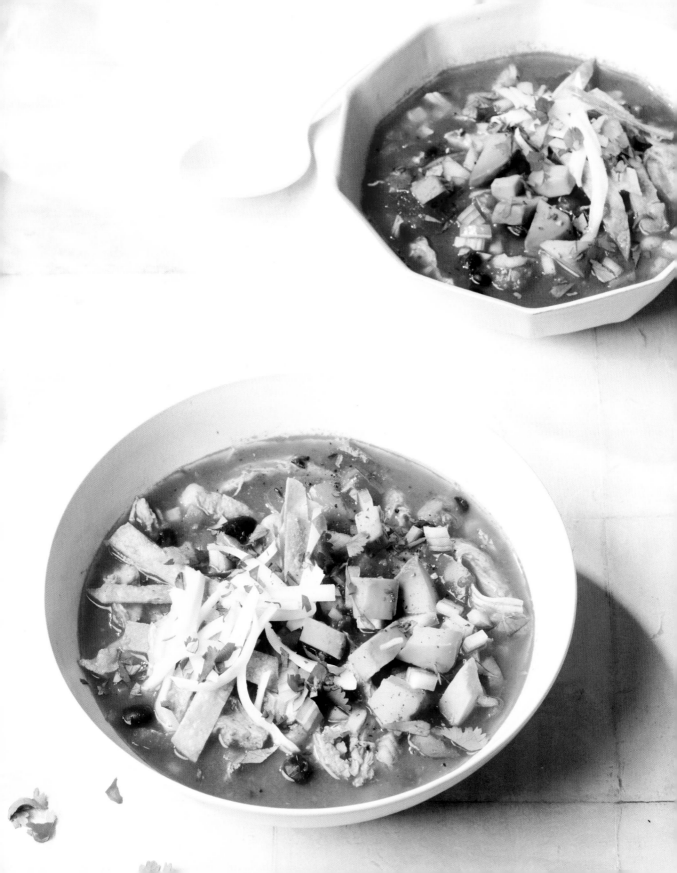

Preheat the oven to 400°F.

In a small bowl, combine all of the spices for the taco seasoning mix and mix together. Set aside.

Spray a rimmed baking sheet with cooking spray or line with parchment paper. Lay the chicken breasts on the baking sheet and sprinkle each side with 2 tablespoons of the taco seasoning mix. Bake for 15 to 20 minutes, until they reach an internal temperature of 165°F. Allow the chicken to cool, then use two forks to shred it. Set aside and reduce the oven temperature to 350°F.

If making your own crispy tortilla strips, arrange the tortilla slices on a large baking sheet sprayed with cooking spray. Bake until the strips are golden and crisp, about 15 minutes.

While the chicken is cooking, heat a large saucepan over medium-high heat. Add the avocado oil and swirl to coat the bottom of the pan. Add the bell peppers, onion, and garlic and sprinkle with the remaining taco seasoning mix. Cook for 3 to 5 minutes, until the onions are translucent.

Add the crushed tomatoes, tomato paste, black beans, corn, hominy, green chilies, chicken broth, and shredded chicken. Bring the mixture to a boil, reduce the heat to a simmer, and cook for 15 to 20 minutes, until the soup is warmed through and the flavors have melded. Serve sprinkled with the toppings of your choice.

TEX-MEX QUINOA BURGERS

So many veggie burgers just don't deliver the taste or texture you're craving in a burger—which is why Cara developed her own recipe! This Tex-Mex veggie burger is perfectly moist thanks to the quinoa and packed with plant-based goodness. It's a balanced meal in a single delicious patty, though feel free to add it to a bun and load it up with all your favorite toppings!

Serves 8

⅓ cup rolled oats

1 (15-ounce) can black beans, rinsed and drained

2 to 3 medium baked sweet potatoes, roughly mashed (about 3 cups)

½ cup cooked quinoa

½ cup frozen sweet corn kernels, thawed

½ cup finely chopped red onion

1 (4-ounce) can diced green chilies

2 tablespoons almond meal or flax meal

1½ tablespoons taco seasoning mix (see page 251)

1 large egg, beaten

Sea salt and freshly ground black pepper

8 slices of your favorite cheese (optional)

8 whole grain hamburger buns or 4 pitas, halved, for serving

Spinach, for serving

Optional toppings:
bean sprouts, sliced tomato, sliced avocado

Preheat the oven to 375°F. Line a large baking sheet with parchment paper and set aside.

In a food processor or high-speed blender, pulse the oats into a flour. Set aside.

In a medium bowl, mash half of the black beans with a fork or potato masher. Add the remainder of the beans and mix to combine. Stir in the mashed sweet potato, quinoa, corn, onion, green chilies, almond meal or flax meal, taco seasoning, and egg. Fold in the oat flour and season with salt and pepper.

Using your hands, form the mixture into 8 burger patties. Arrange them on the prepared baking sheet, spacing them evenly. Bake for about 30 minutes, flipping them halfway through, until the patties are browned and cooked through. If making cheeseburgers, place a slice of cheese on top of each patty during the last 5 minutes of cooking.

To serve, create a bed of spinach on each bottom bun or in each pita pocket. Top with a burger patty, bean sprouts, tomato and avocado slices, or other favorite toppings.

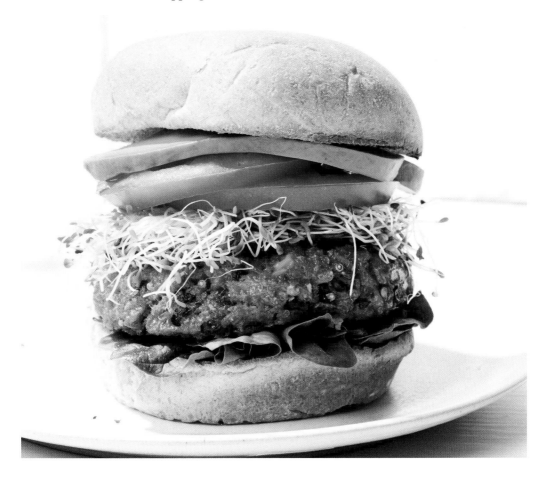

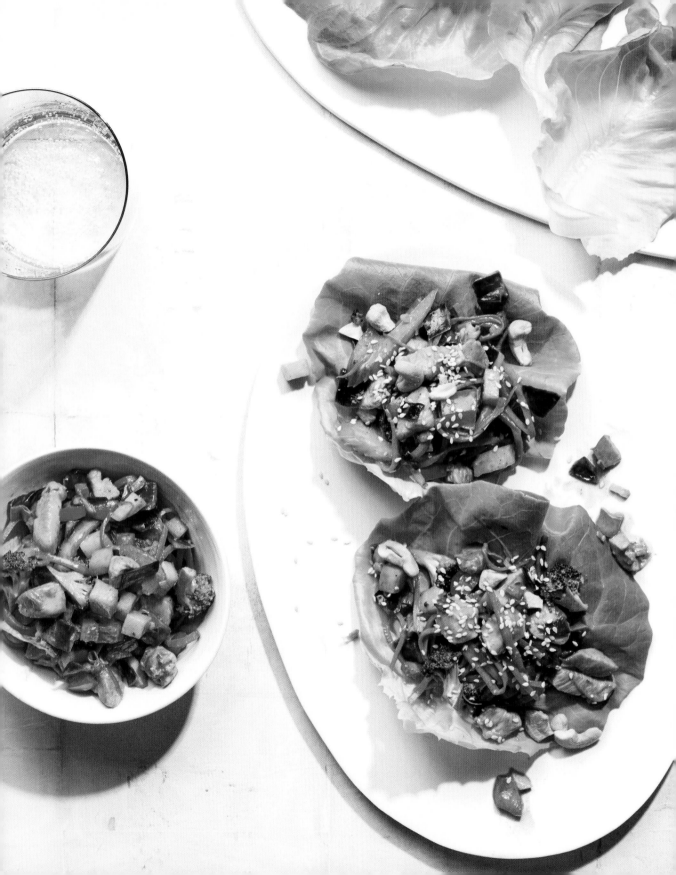

SATAY LETTUCE WRAPS

This is a dish that everyone in the family enjoys—which is saying a lot! You can use ground turkey or chicken here, or swap in a vegetarian protein of your choice. If there happen to be any leftovers, serve them over a bed of greens for lunch the next day.

Serves 4 to 6

For the satay sauce:

⅓ cup plus 1 tablespoon coconut aminos

3 tablespoons natural almond butter

1 tablespoon raw honey or pure maple syrup

2 teaspoons toasted sesame oil

¼ to ½ teaspoon sriracha hot sauce, to taste

For the filling:

1 pound lean ground chicken or ground turkey breast

1 red bell pepper, cored, seeded, and chopped

1 cup finely chopped broccoli

1 cup chopped purple cabbage

1 cup shredded carrots

8 green onions (white and green parts), chopped

½ cup chopped jicama

½ cup chopped celery

For serving:

4 to 6 lettuce leaves (Bibb, Boston, or romaine), washed and dried well

½ cup unsalted cashew pieces

Toasted sesame seeds or hemp seeds

TO MAKE THE SAUCE: In a small bowl or medium jar, whisk or shake together the sauce ingredients until well combined. Set aside.

TO MAKE THE FILLING: In a large nonstick skillet over medium-high heat, cook the meat until browned and no longer pink, 5 to 10 minutes. Add the vegetables and the sauce mixture and cook until the green onions and red peppers are softened and the meat has soaked up the mixture, about 5 minutes more. Remove the pan from the heat.

Spoon about ⅓ cup of the filling into a lettuce leaf. Sprinkle with the cashews and sesame or hemp seeds and enjoy!

CAMPFIRE PACKETS

This is what we call a win-win for family din din. Just assemble your family's favorite veggies plus a lean protein like chicken, chicken sausage, fish, or even beans; then let everyone assemble their own packets to cook in the oven "campfire"-style. No one can complain because they made their own selections, and there's no cleanup afterward. Does it get any better?!

Serves 4

1 pound skinless, boneless chicken breasts, cut into cubes (or chicken sausage, fish, or chickpeas)

1 medium yellow onion, diced

2 bell peppers (color of your choice), cored, seeded, and diced

2 cups cauliflower florets

2 medium carrots, chopped

1 cup snap peas

3 red potatoes, diced

3 sweet potatoes, diced

Kosher salt and freshly ground black pepper

Herbs and spices for seasoning (I love blends like Trader Joe's 21 Seasoning Salute and Mrs. Dash's Salt-Free Seasoning Blend)

Avocado oil, for drizzling

Preheat the oven to 400°F.

Tear off four 8-inch x 8-inch pieces of foil. Then tear off equal-sized squares of parchment paper to lay over each piece of foil (to avoid any toxins from the foil getting into your food).

Create an assembly line by placing all the prepped veggies in individual bowls.

Invite everyone to pile up their desired vegetables onto their piece of foil. Lay the proteins over the top, sprinkle everything with salt and pepper and any other seasonings you like, and give it all a drizzle of avocado oil.

Tightly wrap up each foil parcel and bake for 20 minutes. Unwrap the packets and eat directly from them or transfer the contents to plates.

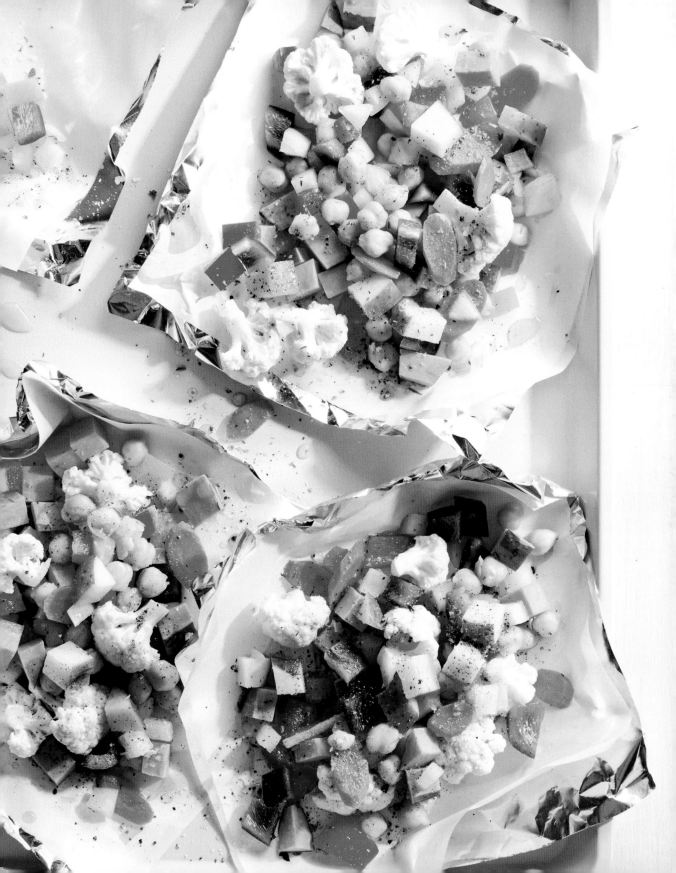

BBQ CHICKEN-STUFFED PEPPERS

Stuffed peppers may seem retro, but we are bringing this week-night staple back into fashion. These peppers are filling, delicious, and packed with all the good things your body needs to thrive. The various colors of bell peppers each have slightly different flavors, with yellow and orange peppers tasting a bit sweeter and red peppers having a little more bite. Choose an array of colors for the prettiest presentation!

Serves 4 to 6

4 bell peppers (red, yellow, or orange), cored and seeded

2½ tablespoons avocado oil

1 cup diced zucchini

1 small yellow onion, chopped

½ jalapeño, minced (seeds removed if you prefer less heat)

3 garlic cloves, minced

1 pound ground chicken breast

Kosher salt and freshly ground black pepper

2 cups chopped spinach or baby spinach leaves

1 cup cooked or canned cannellini beans, rinsed and drained

2 cups cooked quinoa

¾ cup clean BBQ sauce, like Primal Kitchen

1 cup shredded Mexican cheese blend

Preheat the oven to 425°F.

Drizzle the bell peppers with ½ tablespoon of the oil and place them on a baking pan. Roast for 15 minutes, or until the peppers are just tender but not too soft.

Meanwhile, heat the remaining 2 tablespoons oil in a large skillet over medium-high heat. Add the zucchini, onion, jalapeño, and garlic and cook until the zucchini is tender and the onion is translucent, 5 to 6 minutes. Add the chicken, season with salt and pepper, and brown the meat while breaking it up with a spoon or spatula. Fold in the spinach and the beans and sauté until the spinach is wilted, 2 to 3 minutes. Add the quinoa, season with a bit more salt and pepper, then stir in the BBQ sauce. Remove the pan from the heat.

Generously stuff the peppers with the quinoa filling, top each pepper with cheese, and bake for 15 minutes, or until the peppers are completely soft. Switch the oven to broil and finish the peppers under the broiler until the cheese is bubbly and browned, 1 to 2 minutes.

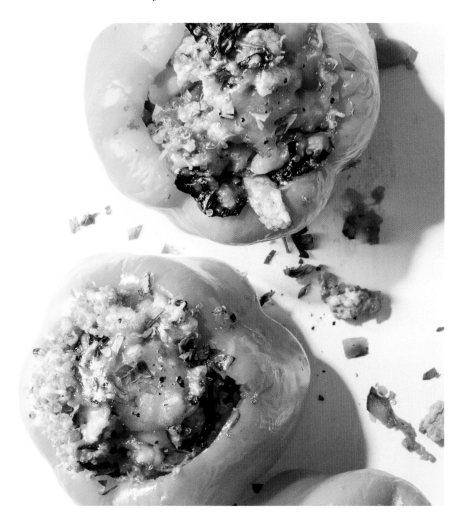

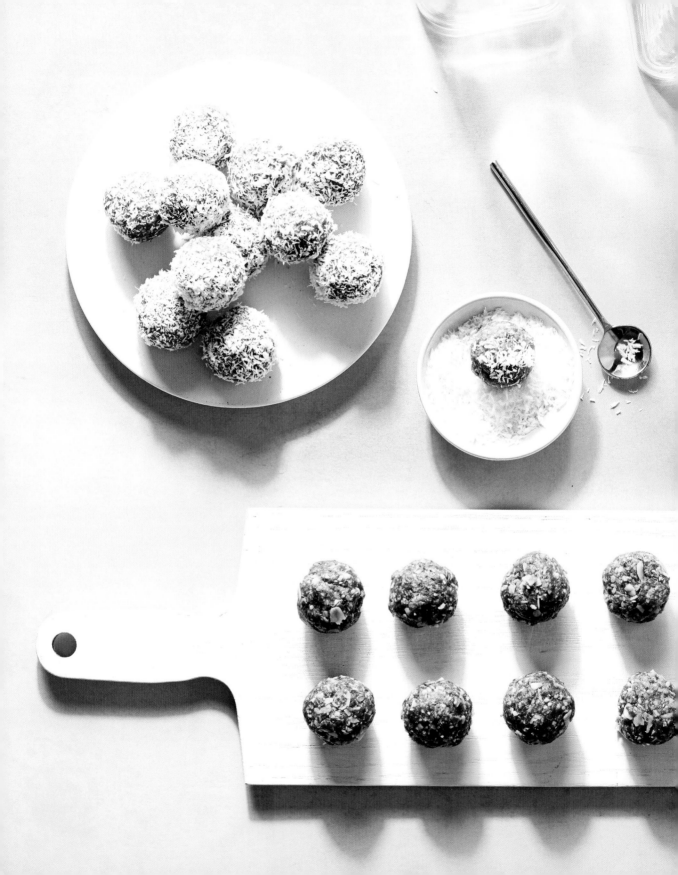

Desserts

COCONUT-LIME ENERGY BITES

These energy bites not only hit the spot for something sweet, they're also nutrient-dense and hit all your macros, thanks to the healthy fats from the coconut and macadamias or cashews, the carbohydrates from the oats, and the protein of the chia and hemp seeds. If you choose to add an algae powder such as spirulina or chlorella, they become even more supercharged with antioxidant and anti-inflammatory powers.

Makes 28 to 30 bites

1 cup pitted dates

1 cup rolled oats

1 cup unsweetened shredded coconut or coconut flakes, plus extra for rolling

½ cup macadamia nuts or cashews

¼ cup hemp seeds

2 tablespoons white chia seeds (black chia are okay, too)

2 tablespoons unsweetened cashew butter

Zest and juice of 2 limes

1 teaspoon pure vanilla extract

½ teaspoon spirulina or chlorella powder (optional)

½ teaspoon maca powder (optional)

¼ teaspoon kosher salt

In a food processor, combine all of the ingredients and pulse until the mixture is evenly chopped and beginning to stick together and form a

(cont.)

ball. Transfer the "dough" to a medium bowl and chill in the refrigerator for 30 minutes.

Using a small ice cream scoop, or about ½ tablespoon measure, portion the dough into balls. Roll each ball with your hands to make it smooth.

Sprinkle shredded coconut or coconut flakes onto a plate and roll the balls in it to lightly coat. Store the bites in an airtight container in the fridge for up to 2 weeks or the freezer for up to 1 month.

OATMEAL COOKIE ENERGY BITES

These "cookies" are a perfect snack or dessert that are super fill-ing, so you won't be tempted to overindulge. I especially love the warm spice that the cardamom lends, combined with the subtle sweetness of the raisins. But if you're really looking for something indulgent, feel free to replace the raisins with dark chocolate chips. Just fold them in after you've mixed together the other ingredients.

Makes about 22 bites

¾ cup raisins

¾ cup plus 3 tablespoons rolled oats

¼ cup pitted Medjool dates

¼ cup unsweetened cashew butter or any other seed/nut butter

¼ cup unsweetened coconut flakes

2 tablespoons flax meal

2 tablespoons hemp seeds

2 teaspoons ground cinnamon

1 teaspoon ground cardamom

1 teaspoon pure vanilla extract

¼ cup raw almonds

¼ cup raw walnuts

¼ teaspoon sea salt

In a food processor, combine all of the ingredients, reserving 3 table-spoons of the oats. Pulse until everything is well mixed and somewhat crumbly. Pour the mixture into a medium bowl and add the reserved oats, stirring until well combined.

Using a small ice cream scoop, or about ½ tablespoon measure, portion the dough into balls. Roll each ball with your hands to make it smooth. Store the bites in an airtight container in the fridge for up to 2 weeks or in the freezer for up to 1 month.

BANANA CHOCO CHIP BLENDER MUFFINS

All of our muffin recipes can be made ahead and stored at room temperature for a week's worth of breakfast and snacks, or frozen and defrosted as desired. These chocolatey muffins satisfy all three macros and deliver two different colors thanks to the banana and zucchini.

Makes about 12 standard-sized muffins or 18 mini muffins

Coconut oil, for greasing (if not using muffin liners)

1½ cups oat flour

2 tablespoons flax meal

2 tablespoons chia seeds

1 teaspoon ground cinnamon

¼ teaspoon ground nutmeg

2 teaspoons baking powder

½ teaspoon baking soda

¼ teaspoon sea salt

2 large bananas

2 eggs (or 2 flax/chia eggs)

2 teaspoons pure vanilla extract

¼ cup plus 2 tablespoons pure maple syrup

¼ cup plus 2 tablespoons sunflower seed butter

1 cup shredded and squeezed dry zucchini (about 1/2 large zucchini)

½ cup dark chocolate chips

Preheat the oven to 350°F. Line 1 mini muffin tin or 2 standard muffin tins with muffin liners or lightly grease them with coconut oil. Set aside.

In a food processor or high-speed blender, pulse the oats into a flour. Add the remaining ingredients except the zucchini and chocolate chips. Blend until everything is well mixed. Transfer the mixture to a medium bowl and fold in the zucchini and chocolate chips.

Divide the batter among the prepared muffins cups, filling them about three-quarters full. Bake for 20 to 25 minutes, until a toothpick or knife inserted in the center comes out clean. Allow the muffins to cool for 10 minutes, then transfer them to a wire rack to cool completely. Store the muffins in an airtight container in the fridge for up to 1 week or freeze them for up to 1 month.

HOMEMADE VANILLA-CINNAMON PECAN BUTTER

We'd just like to say two words about this spread: you're welcome. This life-changing sweet dip is perfect for serving with fruit for an after-school snack or packed up in lunches, or hiding away for a rainy day when you just need a scoop of something good. Just remember that nuts are super nutrient-dense, so a little of this goes a long way! A tablespoon is plenty for getting a beneficial boost.

Makes 2 cups

2 cups pecans, raw or lightly toasted

1 teaspoon ground cinnamon, plus more as needed

½ teaspoon pure vanilla extract

Pinch of sea salt, plus more as needed

In a food processor or high-speed blender, process the pecans until creamy. Pause periodically to scrape down the sides of the blender with a spatula. The texture will be crumbly at first, but as the natural oils release, the mixture will get smooth. Blending time will depend on your individual machine.

Add the cinnamon, vanilla, and salt. Blend again, taste, and add more salt or cinnamon, if desired. Transfer to a pint-sized mason jar and store in the refrigerator for up to 1 week or the freezer for up to 1 month.

ALMOND BUTTER BROWNIES

This is the treat that Christina used to ask for instead of birthday cake—she loves it that much. These dense, gooey brownies are flourless, with almond butter serving as the binder that holds them together. Feel free to play around with this recipe, swapping in different sweeteners (like maple syrup) or nut butters to create your own must-have favorite!

Serves 12

Nonstick coconut oil cooking spray

2 large eggs

1/3 cup raw honey

2 tablespoons coconut sugar

2 teaspoons vanilla extract

1 cup unsweetened creamy almond butter

1/4 cup plus 2 tablespoons cacao or unsweetened cocoa powder

1/2 teaspoon baking soda

1/8 teaspoon sea salt

1/3 cup dark chocolate chips or chocolate chunks

Preheat the oven to 325°F. Line an 8-inch x 8-inch baking dish with parchment paper and spray with cooking spray. Set aside.

In a stand mixer fitted with the whisk attachment or with a hand blender in a large bowl, whip the eggs, honey, sugar, and vanilla until thick and pale. Beat in the almond butter until well combined and smooth. Stir in the cacao or cocoa powder, baking soda, and salt, then fold in the chocolate chips or chunks.

Spread the brownie batter evenly into the prepared pan. Bake for 30 to 35 minutes, until a toothpick or knife inserted into the center comes out clean. Allow the brownies to cool completely, then slice into squares.

If you have any leftovers: (a) you're our hero, and (b) store them in an airtight container in the fridge for up to 1 week or the freezer for up to 1 month.

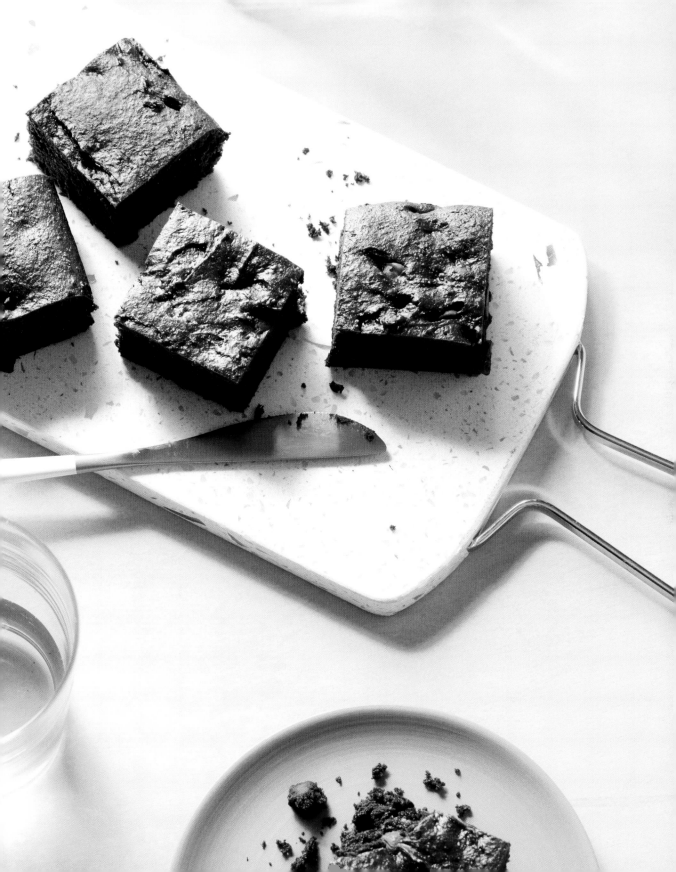

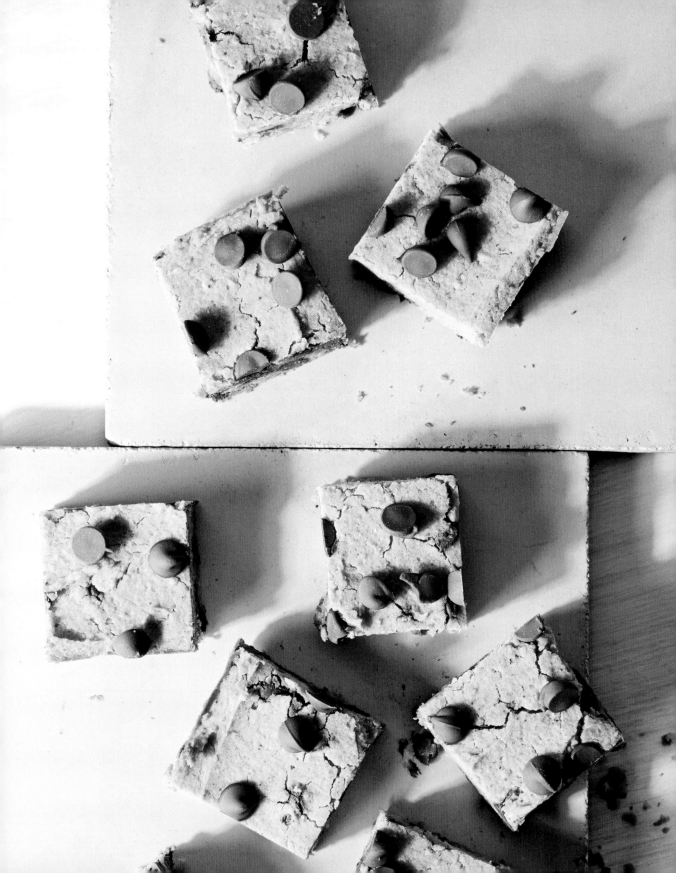

CHICKPEA BLONDIES

These blondies are a huge hit among the foodiest of foodies we know. No one who's tasted one of these rich, buttery, chocolate chip–studded treats has believed that the secret ingredient is chickpeas! What's even better is that these seemingly indulgent squares qualify as a balanced snack thanks to their three macros and no blood sugar–spiking sweeteners. So go ahead and enjoy!

Makes 16 bars

Nonstick coconut oil cooking spray

2 (15-ounce) cans chickpeas, drained and rinsed

¼ cup pure maple syrup

¼ cup honey

¼ cup rolled oats

¼ cup unsweetened creamy almond butter

¼ cup unsweetened creamy peanut butter

1 teaspoon pure vanilla extract

¼ teaspoon sea salt

¾ cup dark chocolate chips

Preheat the oven to 325°F. Line an 8-inch x 8-inch baking dish with parchment paper and spray with cooking spray. Set aside.

Combine all of the ingredients except the chocolate chips in a food processor or blender and process until smooth. Use a spoon or spatula to stir in all but 2 tablespoons of the chocolate chips. Pour the batter evenly into the prepared pan and scatter the remaining chocolate chips over the top. Bake for 25 to 30 minutes, until the blondies have just begun to brown around the edges and are set in the middle. Let them cool in the pan for 10 minutes before slicing. They will last in the fridge for up to 1 week.

BLACK BEAN BROWNIES

These insanely luscious brownies are right up there with our Chickpea Blondies—dense, fudgy, sweet, and not even close to re-sembling an ingredient you'd add to a salad. With a double hit of chocolate in the form of cacao powder and chocolate chips, they satisfy even the most intense chocolate cravings!

Serves 8

Coconut oil cooking spray

1½ cups black beans (one 15-ounce can, drained and rinsed very well)

½ cup quick-cooking oats

½ teaspoon baking powder

2 tablespoons cacao powder

¼ teaspoon kosher salt

½ cup pure maple syrup

¼ cup coconut oil

2 teaspoons pure vanilla extract

⅓ cup dark or semisweet chocolate chips, plus more for sprinkling, if desired

Preheat the oven to 350°F. Line an 8-inch x 8-inch baking dish with parchment paper and spray with cooking spray. Set aside.

In a food processor, combine all of the ingredients except the chocolate chips and process until completely smooth. (A blender will work here if necessary, but the texture and flavor will be better if the mixture gets as smooth and incorporated as possible.)

Transfer the mixture to a medium bowl and fold in the chocolate chips. Pour the batter evenly into the prepared pan and sprinkle with additional chocolate chips, if desired. Bake for 15 to 18 minutes, until the brownies have just begun to brown around the edges and are set in the middle. Let them cool in the pan for 10 minutes, then slice into squares. If they still look a little "fudgy" in the middle, you can place them in the fridge for an hour or up to overnight to firm up. They will last in the fridge for up to 1 week.

PUMPKIN CHOCOLATE CHIP BARS

You don't need to wait until the fall to try these bars, which get their moisture from canned pumpkin—they are delicious all year round. These rich, dense bars are packed with vitamin A, minerals, and fiber from the pumpkin, plus some omega-3s from the chia seeds. This is a go-to recipe for parties and school bake sales—everyone will ask for the recipe!

Serves 12

Coconut oil, for greasing

1½ cups rolled oats

1 cup canned pumpkin puree
  (NOT pumpkin pie filling)

¼ cup raw honey

¼ cup pure maple syrup

¼ cup organic brown sugar

¼ cup organic coconut oil

¼ cup unsalted butter,
  softened

2 large eggs

2 teaspoons pure vanilla extract

¼ cup coconut flour

2 tablespoons chia seeds

1½ teaspoons pumpkin pie spice

1 teaspoon baking soda

¼ teaspoon sea salt

⅓ cup chocolate chips

¼ cup pepitas or hulled
  pumpkin seeds, crushed

Preheat the oven to 350°F. Lightly grease a 9-inch x 13-inch glass baking dish or roasting pan with the coconut oil and set aside.

In a food processor or high-speed blender, pulse the oats into a flour. Set aside.

In a large bowl, combine the pumpkin, honey, maple syrup, sugar, oil, butter, eggs, and vanilla. Mix until the mixture is smooth and creamy, 1 to 2 minutes.

(cont.)

In a separate large bowl, mix together the oat flour, coconut flour, chia seeds, pumpkin pie spice, baking soda, and salt.

Slowly mix the wet ingredients into the dry, stirring until they're just combined. Fold in the chocolate chips.

Pour the batter into the prepared pan and sprinkle the crushed pumpkin seeds over the top. Bake for 20 minutes, or until a toothpick or knife inserted in the center comes out clean. Allow to cool slightly, transfer to a wire rack to cool completely, then slice into bars. Store the bars in an airtight container in the fridge for up to 1 week or the freezer for up to 1 month.

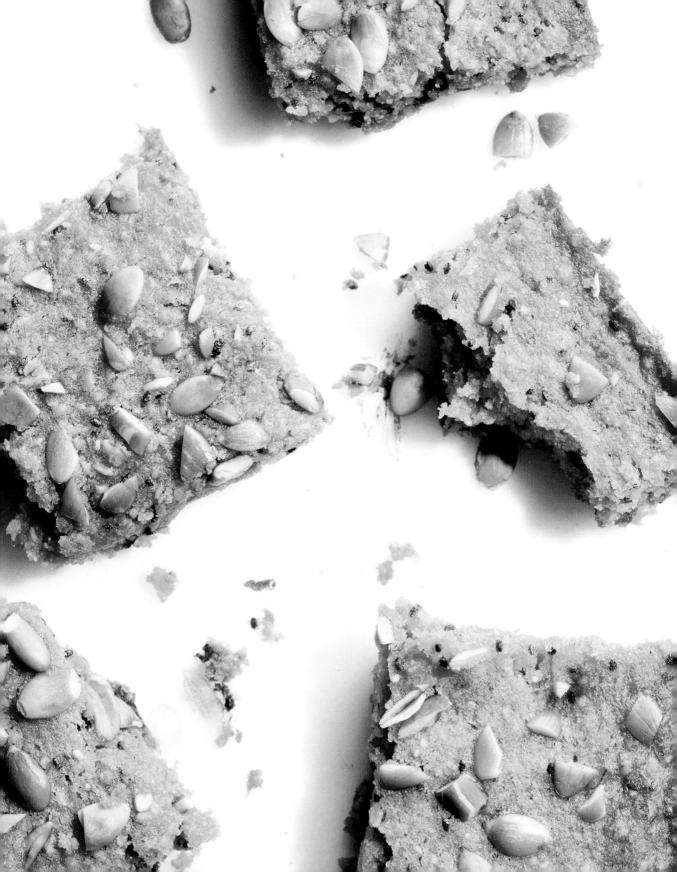

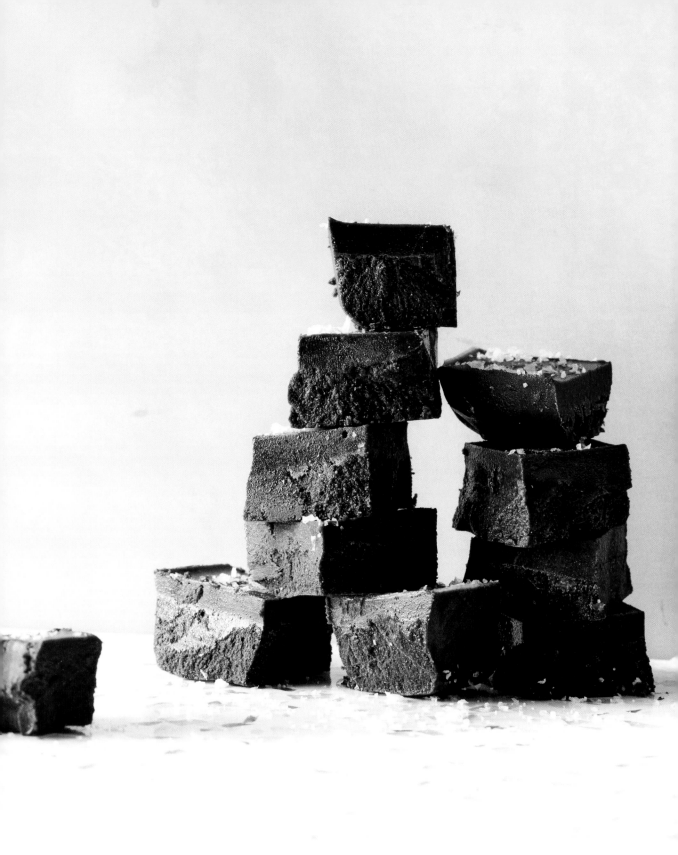

DARK CHOCOLATE SEA SALT FREEZER FUDGE

This recipe needs no introduction because your mouth is probably watering just from the title. And this super-simple fudge 100 percent lives up to its name! It also delivers healing antioxidant properties thanks to the cacao powder, which is the less processed version of cocoa powder. Cacao powder is made from cold-pressing the unroasted cacao beans, which preserves their living enzymes while also maintaining their deep, chocolate flavor. They're basically interchangeable in most recipes, so if you buy a bag, you'll find plenty of ways to put it to good use.

Makes 16 to 20 (1-inch) pieces

1 cup unsweetened creamy almond butter

⅓ cup coconut oil

½ cup unsweetened cacao powder

3 tablespoons raw honey

1 teaspoon pure vanilla extract

Coarsely ground pink Himalayan salt for dusting (try different gourmet flavor varieties for a fun twist!)

Line a 9-inch x 5-inch loaf pan with parchment or wax paper.

In a medium bowl, combine the almond butter and coconut oil. Heat in the microwave for about 30 seconds to warm the mixture, then stir until smooth. You could also do this in a heatproof bowl over a small pot of simmering water. Add the cacao powder, honey, and vanilla. Stir until thoroughly mixed and no clumps remain.

Pour the mixture into the prepared pan and dust with salt. Freeze for at least 2 hours, until completely set. Use the edges of the paper to help lift the fudge out of the pan. Transfer the fudge to a cutting board and slice into 1-inch squares. Enjoy immediately—or at least in the next 15 to 20 minutes, before it begins to melt—or store in an airtight container in the freezer for up to 1 month.

GREEK YOGURT PUMPKIN CHEESECAKE

This recipe is perfect for the holidays, when it can be difficult to find healthy yet satisfying treats that are impressive enough for special family gatherings. This cake not only looks beautiful on a dessert spread and tastes just as good as it sounds, but it also calls for nutrient-dense ingredients, including pumpkin puree, pecans, and almonds. You can also use the nut-honey crust for another cake or pie recipe, or keep leftovers to crumble over yogurt like granola.

Makes one 9-inch pie (serves 8 to 10)

For the crust:
Nonstick cooking spray
1¼ cups almonds
1¼ cups pecans
2 tablespoons raw honey, warmed
Pinch of sea salt

For the filling:
2 cups 2 percent plain Greek yogurt

2 cups pumpkin puree
   (NOT pumpkin pie filling)
6 ounces cream cheese,
   at room temperature
¼ cup plus 1 tablespoon
   raw honey, warmed
2 large eggs
2 teaspoons pure
   vanilla extract
¼ teaspoon ground cinnamon

Preheat the oven to 350°F. Grease a 9-inch pie pan with cooking spray. Set aside.

In a food processor, pulse the almonds and pecans a few times so they are crumbled but not powdery. You could also place them in a plastic zip-top bag and use a mallet or the back of a small pan.

In a medium bowl, combine the crushed nuts with the honey and salt and mix well. Firmly press the mixture into the bottom of the prepared pie pan. It can be helpful to put a piece of wax or parchment paper over the filling to help you get the filling in a nice even layer. (It won't stick to the paper.) Bake for 15 minutes, or until lightly golden. Set aside.

Prepare the filling by first filling a large baking dish or deep-sided pan with water and placing it on the bottom rack of the oven. This will create moisture in the oven, which will prevent the cheesecake from cracking.

In the bowl of a stand mixer fitted with the paddle attachment or in a large bowl with an electric mixer, combine the filling ingredients. Pour the filling over the crust and bake for 50 minutes, or until the edges start to pull away from the sides of the pan and a toothpick or knife inserted into the center comes out clean. Allow the cheesecake to cool at room temperature for at least 30 minutes, then chill in the fridge for 1 hour to set before serving.

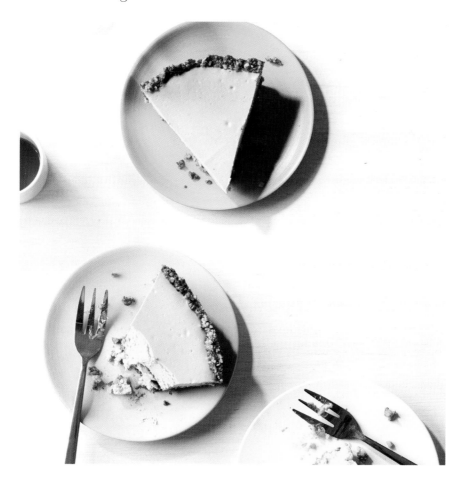

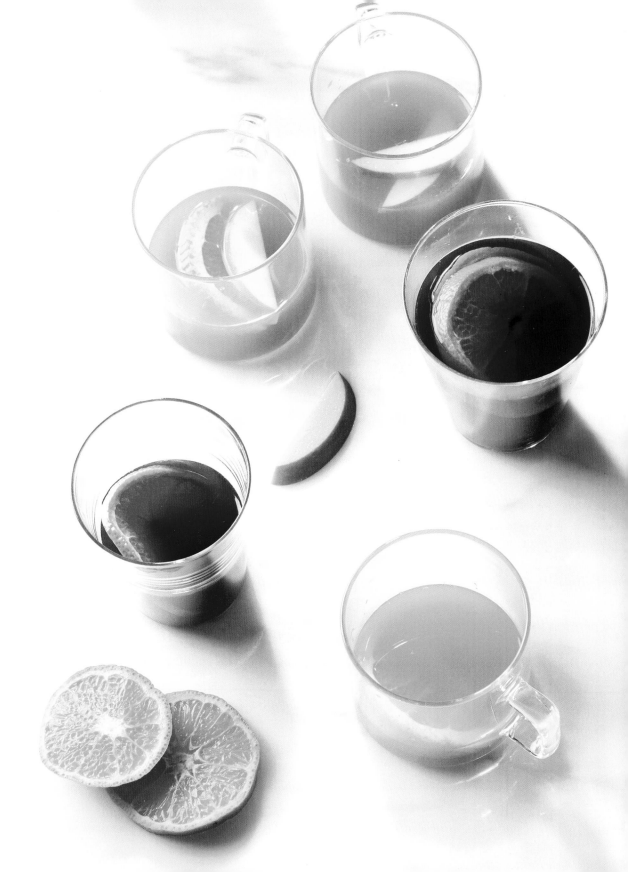

Cocktails

This is a fun batch cocktail that allows you to put your slow cooker to good use (but if you don't have one, no worries, a Dutch oven on the stove works, too). The added bonus of making this festive drink? By the time it's ready your whole house will smell amazing. You can use any red wine blend that's medium dry, though organic versions are best, as they have fewer additives.

Serves 8

1 quart organic unfiltered apple cider

1 bottle of your favorite red blend wine

Juice of 1 lemon

2 clementines, peeled and segmented

½ apple (any type), cored and diced

8 organic mulling spice tea bags

5 cinnamon sticks

In a slow cooker, combine all of the ingredients and set the machine to low or warm. Let the mixture steep for a few hours (ideal for really infusing the flavors). Or you could do this more quickly by bringing the mixture to a simmer on the stovetop and letting the mulling spices steep for at least 15 minutes.

CRANBERRY LIME MOSCOW MULE

The Moscow Mule is the perfect refreshing summer drink. This version uses a splash of cranberry juice, which when combined with the lime is bright and cool, especially on a hot afternoon. And adding a sprig of fresh rosemary plus a small handful of cranberries as garnish makes this a beautiful cocktail for entertaining, too. It's also just as delicious enjoyed as a mocktail.

Serves 1

2 ounces top-shelf vodka or gin
(omit for mocktail version)

1 ounce cranberry juice

1 (12-ounce) bottle ginger beer
(nonalcoholic for mocktail version)

2 lime wedges

1 sprig rosemary, for garnish
(optional)

Fresh or frozen cranberries,
for garnish (optional)

Fill a copper mug (or a mug of your choice) with ice and top with the vodka or gin and cranberry juice. Top off with the ginger beer and a squeeze of lime. Give the mixture a stir and garnish with the lime wedges and the rosemary and cranberries, if desired.

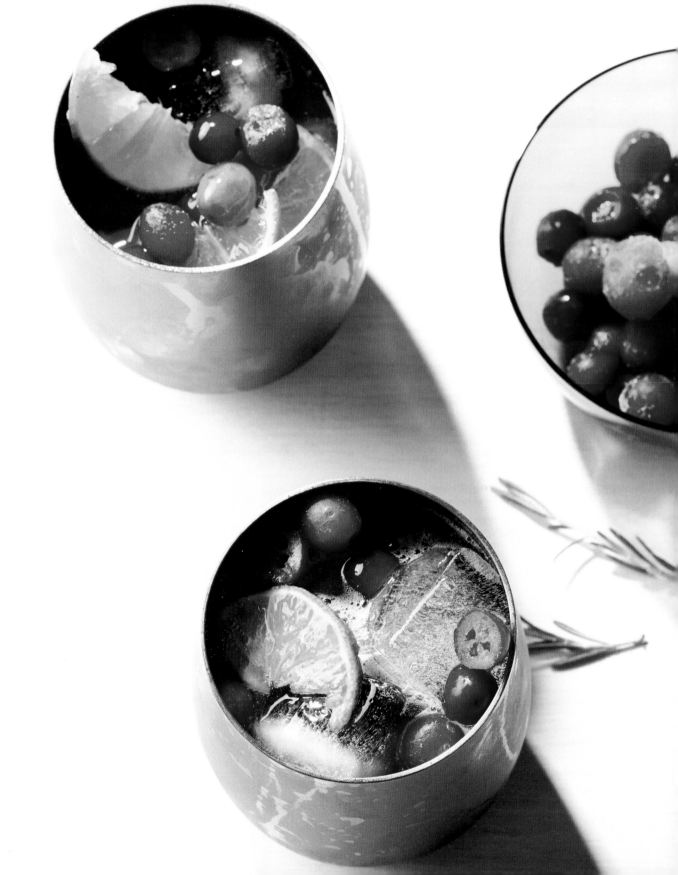

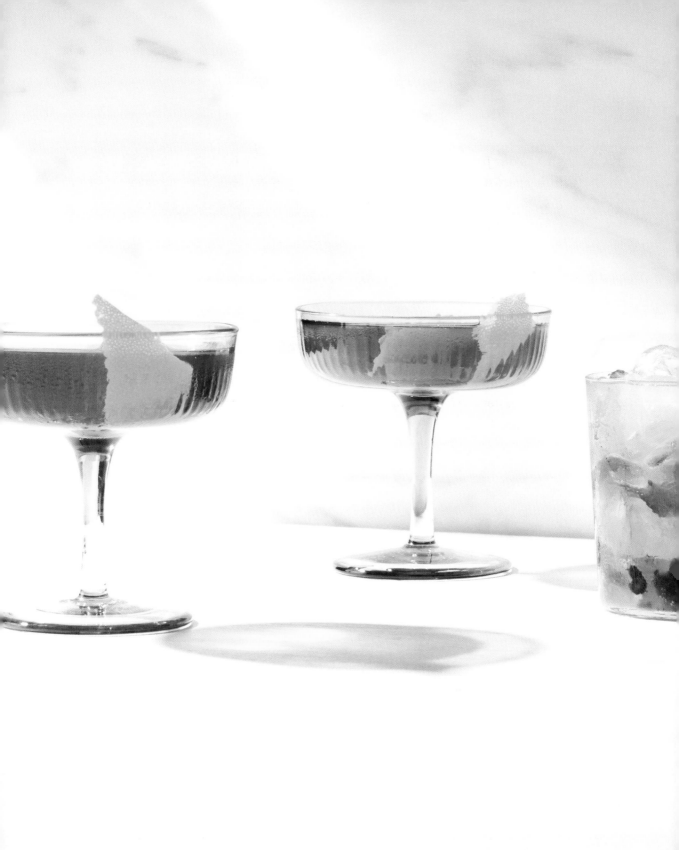

MANHATTAN

This is our fresh, healthy spin on a classic, to which we've added a little sparkling water to lighten things up. You'll feel city-slick with this cocktail in hand, whether you're hosting company or on your couch waiting for the kids to fall asleep.

Serves 1

1 shot whiskey

½ shot vermouth

1 to 2 dashes of bitters

½ cup sparkling water

Orange peel

Pour the whiskey and vermouth in a glass; add a large ice cube and stir. Add the bitters and sparkling water and stir again. Garnish with the orange peel.

BLACKBERRY BOURBON SMASH

Smashing or muddling fresh fruit into your cocktail is an easy way to infuse fresh flavor into your drinks, plus fruit pulp retains anti-oxidant properties, which helps ease the toxic load that alcohol creates in the body. And when it comes to supporting immune health, fresh berries and citrus are high on the list. A splash of ginger kombucha adds spicy flavor while delivering a hit of probiotics.

Serves 1

2 lime wedges

1 lemon wedge

6 fresh blackberries

2 sprigs mint or basil

Handful of ice

1½ ounces top-shelf bourbon (Basil Hayden's is my favorite)

1 (12-ounce) bottle ginger kombucha or ginger beer

In the bottom of a glass, squeeze 1 of the lime wedges and the lemon wedge. Add 5 of the blackberries and 1 mint or basil sprig and muddle (the handle end of a spatula or wooden spoon works well for this if you don't have a muddler). Fill the glass with ice and pour in the bourbon. Top off with the ginger kombucha or beer. Stir and garnish with a blackberry, lime wedge, and sprig of mint.

TEQUILA CITRUS

While all alcohol is received by the body as a toxin, some spirits are easier to process than others. Clear liquors, like vodka and tequila—which is derived from the agave plant—tends to be the gentlest on your system. It has even been suggested that tequila has healing properties! While I'm not doing a shot of tequila to stay healthy, I am reaching for it when I want to make a fun cocktail that isn't going to slow me down.

Serves 1

1½ ounces clear agave tequila

1 cup sparkling water

Juice of ½ grapefruit
  or whole lime

Pour the ingredients over ice and sip.

SPIKED HOT APPLE CIDER

Can't you just see yourself sitting by the fireplace between Thanks-giving and Christmas, reading a good book, and sipping a warm, calming drink? Now you can achieve maximum coziness with this warmly spiced cider, whether you're enjoying a mug on your own or serving it up at your next holiday party.

Serves 6

1 quart unfiltered apple cider

8 cinnamon sticks

1 tablespoon orange zest

1 tablespoon fresh orange juice

1 teaspoon whole cloves

1 teaspoon grated fresh ginger

¼ cup spiced rum or bourbon

Apple slices, for garnish (optional)

In a medium saucepan, combine the apple cider, 2 of the cinnamon sticks, the orange zest, orange juice, cloves, and ginger. Bring the mixture to a boil over high heat, reduce the heat to low, and simmer for 10 minutes. Remove the pot from the heat and strain through a fine-mesh strainer. Discard any solids.

Stir in the rum or bourbon and serve warm, with each mug garnished with the remaining cinnamon sticks and apple slices, if desired.

POMEGRANATE SPRITZER

This pretty pink drink provides inflammation-fighting antioxidants from fresh grapefruit juice and pomegranate arils, which help the body absorb more of what it needs and get rid of what it doesn't. This low-sugar drink is great for those who don't like sweet cocktails—it is refreshingly tart!

Serves 1

¼ cup LaCroix Grapefruit (or other naturally flavored sparkling water)

1½ ounces vodka

2 tablespoons fresh grapefruit juice

20 pomegranate arils

4 fresh mint leaves, for garnish

Combine the sparkling water, vodka, grapefruit juice, and pomegranate arils in a glass over ice. Stir, garnish with the mint leaves, and enjoy.

SKINNY MARGARITA

Okay, let's be real: No drink is going to make you skinny. But if you are going to go for a margarita, this lower-calorie, lower-sugar version is a good choice. It's usually on the menu when we get together with girlfriends!

Serves 1

1 lime, sliced into 4 wedges

1 orange wedge

Handful of ice

1½ ounces top-shelf tequila (such as 1800 or El Jimador Reposado)

½ ounce Grand Marnier

½ teaspoon pure maple syrup (optional)

Lime seltzer

In the bottom of a glass, squeeze 1 of the lime wedges and the orange wedge. Optionally, you could add the entire wedge of each and muddle to release the natural oils from the peels, which have a bright, bitter flavor.

Add ice to fill the glass and pour in the tequila, Grand Marnier, juice of 2 lime wedges, and maple syrup, if using. Stir. Top off with lime seltzer, stir again, and garnish with the remaining lime wedge, and serve.

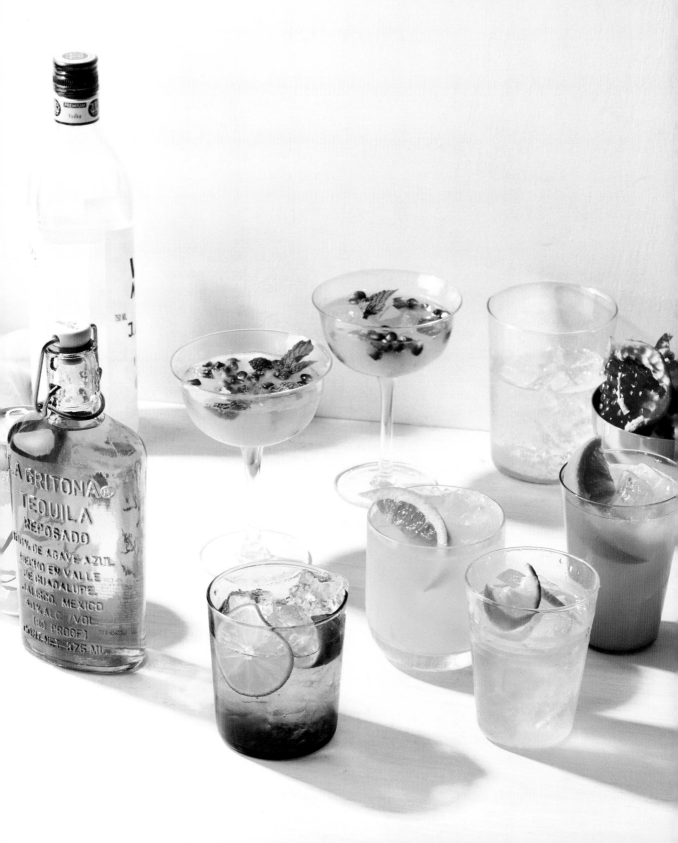

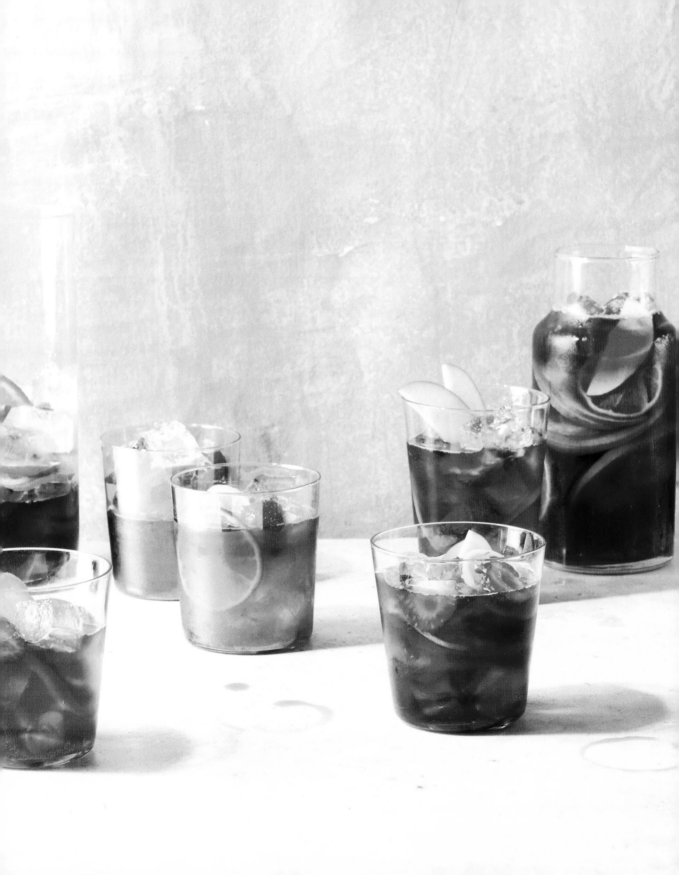

SUMMER SANGRIA

If you're looking for a festive, refreshing drink to serve at your next barbecue or other warm-weather gathering, this is the perfect fit. Not only is this sangria delicious, it's also loaded with antioxidants to offset the effects of the alcohol. Just don't be fooled by how easy it is to drink!

Serves 6

1 bottle of your favorite pinot noir (or other medium/light-bodied red wine)

3 ounces top-shelf brandy or spiced rum

1 can LaCroix Orange or Mango

1 lemon, sliced

1 lime, sliced

1 orange, sliced

4 to 5 strawberries, sliced

½ small apple, sliced or diced

Combine all of the ingredients in a pitcher and serve.

KOMBUCHA VODKA

This cocktail is one we frequently whip up when we want to celebrate but don't have a lot of ingredients on hand. Since we usually keep kombucha stocked in our fridges, all we need to do is add a shot of vodka and voila. Just remember, when making drinks with kombucha—stir, don't shake!

Serves 1

1 cup Trilogy Synergy Kombucha or kombucha of your choice

1 shot vodka

Fresh basil leaf, or other herb, to garnish (optional)

Combine the kombucha and vodka in a glass and stir to combine. Garnish as desired and enjoy.

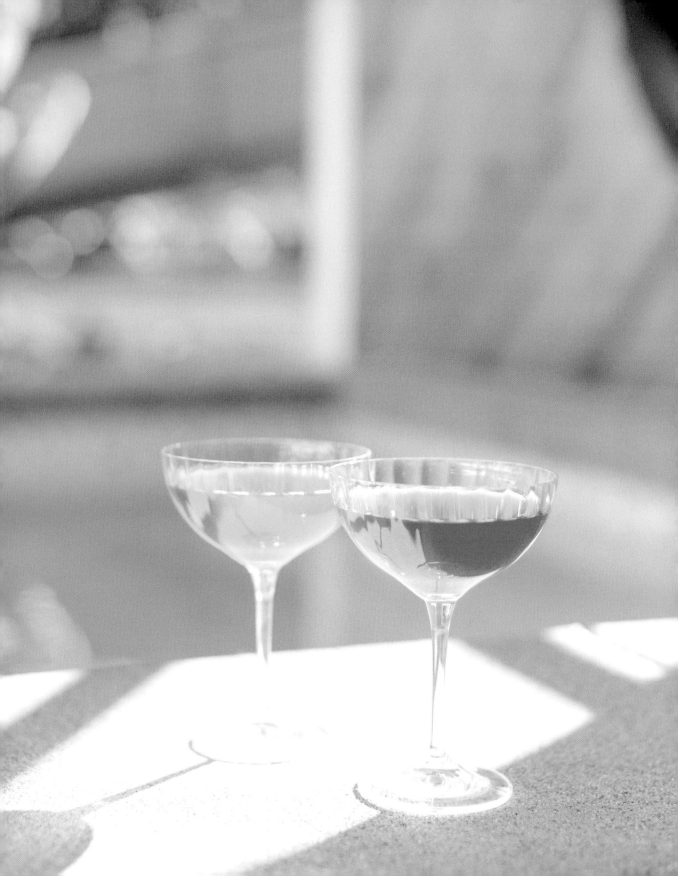

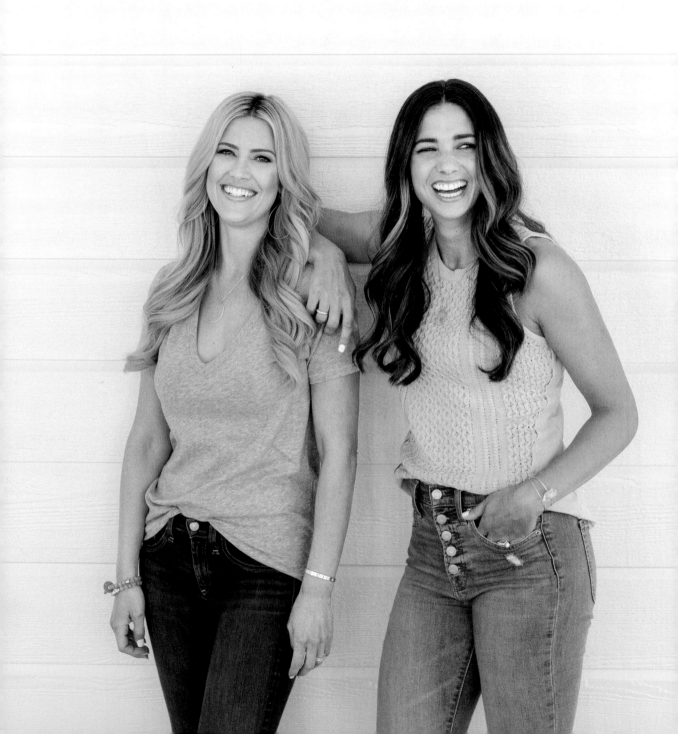

Acknowledgments

In our lives, it literally takes a village to get things done, and this book is no exception. *The Wellness Remodel* has been a collaboration by so many talented people, to whom we owe so many thanks.

From Christina:

To all my faithful followers, I hope you gain some new knowledge and perspective after reading this.

To my attorney and friend, Roger Behle, thank you for your support and guidance throughout the years.

To our literary agent, Todd Shuster, thanks for sticking by my side throughout the years. I look forward to more projects together!

To our editor, Julie Will, thanks for believing in this project!

To the whole crew at HarperCollins, we prayed you would pick us and couldn't be more pleased to do this project with you.

To our collaborator, Rachel Holtzman, thank you for putting our thoughts and ideas onto pages. You are amazing.

To my coauthor, Cara Clark, I'm so grateful to know you—you are a superhero, and I loved doing this project with you. I can't wait to see what the future has in store for us!

To my parents, Paul and Laurie, for always pushing me and teaching me to work hard.

To my talented husband, Ant Anstead, for always encouraging, lifting, and grounding me. Love you always.

To my children Taylor, Brayden, and Hudson, I love being your mom; you each inspire me every day.

From Cara:

I would like to acknowledge:

My coauthor, Christina Anstead: Thank you for trusting me first as your nutritionist and then as your friend. You have pushed me past my self-prescribed limitations, and I'm forever grateful for you. Thank you for being vulnerable in the creation of this book and for sharing some of your most sacred moments in your health journey.

To my Cara Clark Nutrition team: All of you have played a huge part in this book!

Allison Long, you have been the best assistant nutritionist on the planet, and many of these recipes evolved from your kitchen! Thanks for all you have given the CCN community.

Ashlee Thomas, you are my right-hand girl, a godsend truly! Thank you for consistently reading my mind and being open to my crazy ideas.

Lisa Ashton, you believed in me more than anyone else. Thank you for always being there and constantly envisioning new and great ideas for CNN!

Nellie, Amelia, Aubrey: Ladies, we couldn't do this without you! Thank you.

To my parents, Dennis and Mary Busson, you have given me everything in teaching me my faith. You told me that God gave me my talents to help others and here I am. I'm so thankful to you for pushing me, supporting me, and lifting me up with your unconditional love.

To my six siblings, and my brother in heaven: Your prayers and love mean everything to me. Thank you for believing in me. Thank you for teasing me and calling me "fantasy world" because I always wanted to prove to you that my fantasy world could come true.

Last but not least, to the loves of my life: Chris, you have never stopped pushing me, believing in me, and committing to me, to my work, and to us.

I will love you forever! Maggie, Mila, Claire, and Carli, every day you inspire me to be a better person. You challenge me to be more patient and understanding. I am so passionate about nutrition so that you girls have a future that involves food freedom and so you can maybe even help others understand the power of food. The five of you have given me a life beyond my wildest dreams. I love you!

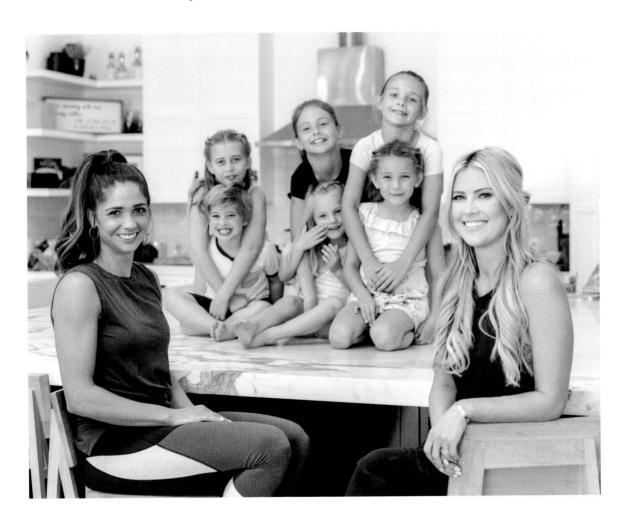

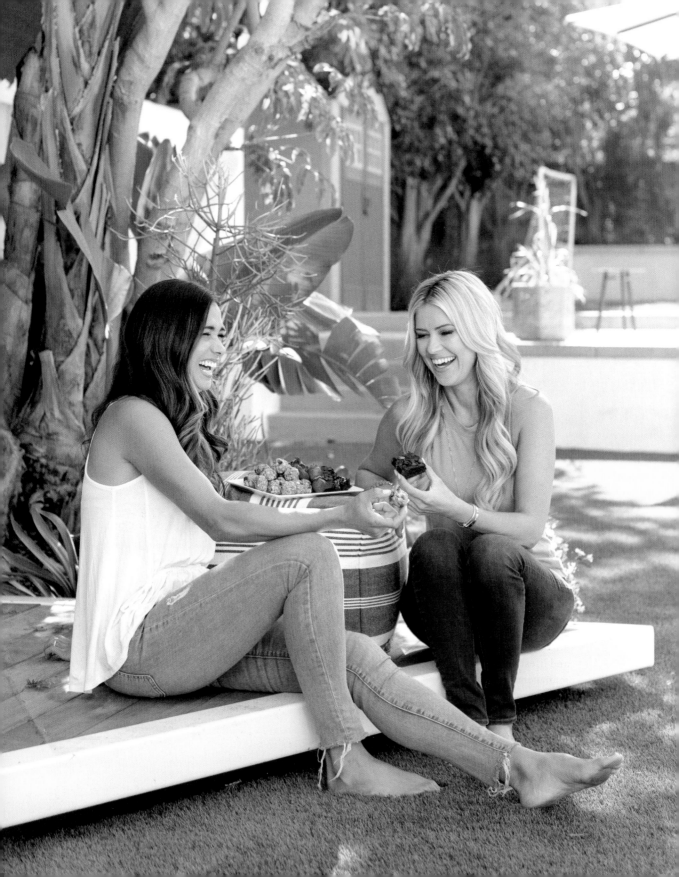

Index

Note: Italic page numbers refer to charts and illustrations.

muffins
Banana Choco Chip Blender Muffins, 266
Good Morning Muffins, 201–2, *202*
Harvest Oat Muffins, 203–4, *205*
Peanut Butter Chia Chocolate Chip Muffins, *218*, 219

negative thinking patterns, 72
neurological system, 70
nut butters, 15, 40, 70–71, 159
nutritional science, 37
nuts and seeds, 27, 28–29, 40, 45, 70–71, 159, 161

Oatmeal Cookie Energy Bites, 265
oats, 159
obesity, lowering chances of, 200
oils, plant-derived oils, 27, 45, 160
olive oil, 15, 44, 160
On Your Marks Fitness, 89
Orangetheory, 78, 83
organized improvisers, meal prep for, 163–64, 179–80

pancakes, Pumpkin-Pecan Pancakes, 192, *193*
pantry staples, 52, *55*, 67, 68, 156, 157–61, 164, 179
parasympathetic nervous system, 125, 126, 133
pasta
as pantry staple, 160

Quick Cannellini & Spinach Pasta, 243
pasta sauce, 160
PB&J Overnight Oats, *198*, 199
Peanut Butter Chia Chocolate Chip Muffins, *218*, 219
phytochemicals, 9, 33
Pilates, 80
Pineapple Stir-Fry, 241
Pinterest, 150, 175
pizza, Breakfast Pizza, 196, *197*
plank reach, 111, *111*
plank toe taps, 114, *114*
plank-walk cleanup, 176
planners
meal prep for, 164–65
new-normal life checklist for, 176–77
plie squats, 101, *101*
polycystic ovary syndrome (PCOS), 4, 8, 13, 123, 125
Pomegranate Spritzer, 289
positive affirmations, 72
potatoes, 24, 227
prediabetes, 19
pregnancies, 13, 16, 123
present moment, focusing on, 122, 133
probiotics, 46–47, 173
processed foods, 15, 25, 32–33, 43
progesterone, 125
protein
function of, 28–29
as macronutrient, 23
pairing with carbohydrates, 21, 23–29, 168
sources of, 28
puddings
Berry Coconut Chia Pudding Parfait, 210

Choco Maca Chia Pudding, 188, *189*
Coconut-Pistachio Chia Pudding, 188, *189*
Pumpkin Chocolate Chip Bars, 273–74, *275*
Pumpkin-Pecan Pancakes, 192, *193*

Quick Cannellini & Spinach Pasta, 243
quinoa, 29, 160
Quinoa Bowl, 237

reading, 133, 140, 147, 173
rebounders, 175
red meat, 16
Reiki, 71
religions, 23. *See also* faith
Remodel hacks
being okay with chaos, 169–74
family involvement, 166, 168–69
fitting daily activity during everyday life, 174–76
getting prepared, 156–61, 163–65
new-normal life checklist, 176–77
pantry staples, 157–61
resistant starches, 24
"rest and digest" mode, 125
restrictive mind-sets, 72–73
rewire, 5–6. *See also* faith; mindfulness practices; spirituality
rice, 160
rice cakes, 160

About the Authors

CHRISTINA ANSTEAD is best known as the cohost of the hit HGTV shows *Flip or Flop* and *Christina on the Coast*. Alongside her busy roles within the property and television sectors, she is a wife and a mama to three beautiful children. Christina is not a wellness expert, but she has lived and learned, and she has become a passionate advocate for leading a balanced lifestyle that supports the mind, body, and spirit.

CARA CLARK is the owner and primary nutritionist of Cara Clark Nutrition. Her philosophy of creating balance and nurturing the whole body has been adopted by over 20,000 households, including those of numerous celebrities and Olympic athletes. Cara is also a certified sports and clinical nutritionist specializing in prenatal and postpartum nutrition and working with performance athletes and individuals with diabetes. She lives in Orange County, California, with her husband and four daughters.

THE WELLNESS REMODEL. Copyright © 2020 by Christina Anstead and Cara Clark. All rights reserved. Printed in the United States of America. No part of this book may be used or reproduced in any manner whatsoever without written permission except in the case of brief quotations embodied in critical articles and reviews. For information, address HarperCollins Publishers, 195 Broadway, New York, NY 10007.

HarperCollins books may be purchased for educational, business, or sales promotional use. For information, please email the Special Markets Department at SPsales@harpercollins.com.

FIRST EDITION

DESIGNED BY BONNI LEON-BERMAN

PHOTOGRAPHY BY ANGELICA VALITON / ANGELICA MARIE PHOTOGRAPHY

Library of Congress Cataloging-in-Publication Data has been applied for.

ISBN 978-0-06-296144-0

33614081700642

20 21 22 23 24   LSC   10 9 8 7 6 5 4 3 2 1

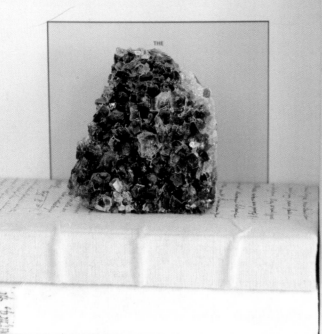

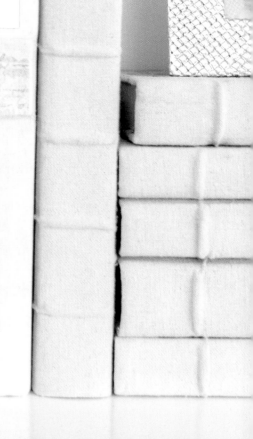